Speech and Language Therapy and Professional Identity

This book is a sum of the "dangling conversations" that we have had over the course of our professional careers to date.

(thanks to Paul Simon)

Speech and Language Therapy and Professional Identity

Challenging received wisdom

Jane Stokes and
Marian McCormick
(Editors)

J&R Press Ltd

© 2015 J&R Press Ltd

All rights reserved. No part of this publication may be reproduced, stored in a retrieval system or transmitted in any form or by any means, electronic, mechanical, photocopying, recording, scanning or otherwise, except under the terms of the Copyright Designs and Patents Act 1988 or under the terms of a licence issued by the Copyright Licensing Agency Ltd, without the permission in writing of the Publisher. Requests to the Publisher should be addressed to J&R Press Ltd, Farley Heath Cottage, Albury, Guildford GU5 9EW, or emailed to rachael_jrpress@btinternet.com.

The use of general descriptive names, registered names, trademarks, etc. in this publication does not imply, even in the absence of a specific statement, that such names are exempt from the relevant protective laws and regulations and therefore free for general use.

Library of Congress Cataloguing in Publication Data
British Library Cataloguing in Publication Data
A catalogue record for this book is available from the British Library
Cover design: Jim Wilkie
Project management, typesetting and design: J&R Publishing Services Ltd, Guildford, Surrey, UK; www.jr-publishingservices.co.uk
Indexed by Terry Halliday (HallidayTerence@aol.com)

Printed and bound by CPI Group (UK) Ltd, Croydon, CR0 4YY

Contents

About the contributors	vii
Introduction	1
1 Reflective practice in speech and language therapy Marian McCormick	17
2 To intervene or not to intervene Aoife Gallagher	43
3 Supervision in speech and language therapy: Learning from other professions Jane Stokes	65
4 Using video to catch, develop and propagate emerging skills with parents, children, educators and therapists Keena Cummins	79
5 A sociocultural perspective on speech and language therapy and education: Overlaps between the two professions Deirdre Martin and Jane Stokes	109
6 Spirituality and speech and language therapy Sophie MacKenzie	127
7 Cultural and linguistic diversity issues in the profession Jane Stokes	143
8 Speech and language therapy and gender Chris Markham and Catherine Neal	157
9 A critical look at the concept of 'service' in speech and language therapy Jane Stokes	181
10 In conclusion Marian McCormick and Jane Stokes	201
Index	213

About the contributors

Keena Cummins started her career as a speech and language therapist working with adults and children, whose impact on her was profound. Keena's observation of the impact of the environment on the people she worked with led her to understand that the power balance of interaction was central to how people accessed and developed their communication, language and learning. Lena Rustin, her manager, placed professional team dynamics and self-reflection at the heart of service delivery. Keena led an early years team, ensuring that video provided each parent with the opportunity to observe their own skills and facilitate the development of their child through confident use of those skills. She introduced a video supervision system for all therapists. She now has an independent practice working with parents and children, and works with video in Early Years settings, Primary and Secondary schools. Her work includes supporting speech and language therapy teams in using video interaction therapy with clients and using video for team supervision and support. She is a visiting lecturer at City University and the University of Greenwich. Her luxury remains the things she learns daily from each child, their parents, their educators and self-reflective professional peers.

Aoife Gallagher qualified as a Speech and Language Therapist in 1996 from Trinity College Dublin. She has worked in different NHS trusts in London, across a range of settings. She did a Masters in Human Communication at the University of London evaluating the effectiveness of different service models for children with specific language impairments. She has managed a multidisciplinary therapy team of SLTs OTs, Physiotherapists for a charity providing assessment and intensive therapy to children and young people with severe specific language impairments. She has worked as a medico-legal expert witness in Special Educational Needs Tribunal Appeals. Since 2013, Aoife has been working at the University of Limerick, currently as a Lecturer. Her research interests include evaluating the effectiveness of different models of intervention and dosage in speech and language therapy.

Sophie MacKenzie graduated in 1990 from City University and has spent the majority of her career working with adults with neurological conditions, especially stroke and head injury. She began working as a senior lecturer in Speech and Language Therapy at the University of Greenwich in 2007, initially combining this with the role of Clinical Manager in Speech and Language Therapy at a local Trust. She now works full time lecturing in adult acquired communication and swallowing disorders at the University of Greenwich and Canterbury Christ Church University, and is director of the post graduate diploma programme in SLT.Sophie is currently undertaking a PhD, exploring the concept of spirituality with people with aphasia.

Chris Markham has been a registered speech and language therapist for 15 years, and has worked within the National Health Service, Local Authorities and Higher Education. During this time Chris has supported clients with a range of communication needs and led research studies within both children's and adult services and the wider field of Health Service Research. Chris is currently employed as an Associate Head of an Academic Health and Social Care Sciences Department, with a particular focus on research and innovation. He continues to teach under and post graduate students and conduct research within the field of the Allied Health Professionals.

Deirdre Martin is Professor of Language, Culture and Learning at Goldsmiths, University of London. Her research concerns disability, and particularly language and literacy disabilities in multilingual families and educational settings. She qualified as a speech and language therapist and has worked through Spanish as a SLT overseas, and with multilingual communities in England. With Jane Stokes and colleagues she contributed to the RCSLT Special Interest Group on Bilingualism and on raising the profile of multilingualism in the profession. She has been involved in major funded research projects, and most recently the Economic and Social Research Council funded Researcher Development Initiative, *Researching Multilingualism: Multilingual research practice*, with Professor Marilyn Martin-Jones. Previously, at the University of Birmingham, she leads two masters programmes: 'Speech and Language Difficulties' and 'Language, Literacies and Dyslexia'. Her publications include: *Language Disabilities in Cultural and Linguistic Diversity* (2009) Bristol: Multilingual Matters; *Researching Dyslexia in Multilingual Settings* (Ed) (2013) Bristol: Multilingual Matters.

Marian McCormick has been a practising SLT for 25 years, in which time she has worked in a variety of settings in the UK, New Zealand and Australia. Until January 2013 she was Programme Director on the Postgraduate Diploma in Speech and Language Therapy at Canterbury Christ Church University. She continues to lecture on the programme and takes a lead on the teaching of reflective practice. Since joining the university in 2006, her interests in learning and teaching and integrating reflective practice into SaLT education have underpinned her work.

Jane Stokes was a practising speech and language therapist for 25 years. For the last 14 years of that period, she was a clinical manager, responsible for managing teams of speech and language therapists working with children, in community settings, schools and Sure Start programmes. Her research interests focus on children from culturally and linguistically diverse groups. She was a visiting lecturer to City University, London, and worked as a clinical tutor supporting speech and language therapy students. In 2006 she took up her current role as senior lecturer on a new postgraduate diploma in speech and language therapy at University of Greenwich. Her work has been influenced and enhanced by the diverse populations with whom she has worked, and the fascinating ongoing collaborations with student practitioners and colleagues across various disciplines in practice and in Higher Education.

Introduction

Speech and language therapy and professional identity: Challenging received wisdom

Jane Stokes and Marian McCormick

> "Walking along a path, in life or in a career, is like a long hike on a challenging trail. It is step by step."
> (Skovholt and Trotter-Mathison, 2011, p. 39)

This book reflects the stories that we have collected along the journey of creating and establishing a new postgraduate programme in speech and language therapy. The metaphor of journey has been a useful one in this process as with each experience the landscape altered, new structures appeared on the horizon, environmental conditions changed and situations occurred that presented challenges that had to be negotiated and overcome. There were twists and turns which could not have been anticipated at the start which required a response, a detour and sometimes a change of direction. So we present this book "… not [as] a record of what happened… but rather as a continuing interpretation and re-interpretation of [our] experience" (Bruner, 1988, p.575).

In delivering the programme, we have felt at times like tour guides introducing new students to the landscape of the profession. We have been in the position of having to show them what organisations such as McKinsey call "how to do things round here". We have designed and delivered a curriculum that has met regulatory requirements and introduced the students to the humanistic philosophic underpinnings, and the legal, ethical and professional frameworks which underpin clinical practice. They have been introduced to the biological sciences and psychological concepts relevant to speech and language therapy; they have learned about linguistics, phonetics, phonology, audiology. In collaboration with colleagues in practice, we have facilitated their learning of reflection, technical and clinical skills; have prepared them for placement learning; encouraged them in their reflective logs; and developed their understanding of communication difficulties in a wide range of contexts. Those were the challenges we knew we would face.

A challenge we had not foreseen was that of introducing the students to the more tacit knowledge embedded within the profession, the prevailing ideological and theoretical perspectives, the unconsciously accepted aspects of professional practice and the culture of the profession. This culture plays a powerful role in determining our professional values and ways of working, it articulates and defines our collective understanding of the profession, and it is from this bedrock that our professional 'received wisdom' has emerged. Through observing and hearing about the experiences of student practitioners as they interact with their chosen career, we have had an opportunity to hold a mirror up to the profession of speech and language therapy in the UK. Many aspects of this process have been intensely rewarding and stimulating; other aspects, however, have resulted in some uncomfortable insights and some unsettling experiences. We have at times struggled to negotiate the tensions between key professional issues, and have come up against some big questions about professional identity, culture and practice. We have had many lively debates with each other and colleagues about dimensions and fundamentals of practice, priorities and preconceptions in preparing students to work in the changing landscape of professional practice.

We have attempted to uncover a few stones that are features of this tacit knowledge in order to look underneath them, but they have been heavy to lift at times. Some of the ideas within the text of this book may present as provocative, controversial or maverick, and some are still just thoughts, yet to be tested widely. We do not claim to be presenting the evidence from methodologically sound research. We are throwing pebbles into the metaphorical pool of professional discourse and, in doing so, we hope to provoke further discussion.

This book aims to:

- Raise some of the unexplored, received wisdom about the role of the speech and language therapist

- Add to the debates about the aims and objectives of the profession, by exploring some of the unspoken sets of values that often surround our work, and questioning what we do and why

- Examine some of the contexts for professional practice that are rarely explored
- Encourage colleagues and future therapists to challenge, question, and adapt, using critical appraisal skills combined with reflective practice.

Central to all of these aims is the question of the nature of professional knowledge, skills and understanding which have to be acquired and demonstrated in the development of professional competence. Tensions exist between the focus on evidence-based practice and the value placed on intuition or practice wisdom, tacit knowledge, and the fact that a considerable amount of practice has no scientific evidential base, in some cases because this evidence has not yet been identified and at times because, at least in principle, some aspects of professional practice can never be understood by the tools of empirical science (Higgs, Richardson and Dahlgren, 2004, p.63).

The nature of knowledge: Defining expertise and competence

Within speech and language therapy as within other health professions there are different kinds of knowledge. Higgs and Titchen (1995) outlined three categories of professional knowledge: **propositional knowledge**, i.e., that which is derived through research and scholarship, and two types of **non-propositional knowledge**: **professional craft knowledge**, embedded in practice, which includes so-called tacit knowledge, or background knowledge shaped from long familiarity with the profession, and **personal knowledge**, derived from an individual's life experiences.

In this next section, we examine more closely the nature of these 'types of knowing' within practice, and how they contribute to, and influence professional culture.

Propositional knowledge: Speech and language therapy and the positivist paradigm

Speech and language therapy is not alone in its heavy reliance on practice wisdom. History and anecdote have formed the basis of much treatment within the health service (Enderby and Emerson, 1995). Everyday practices in social work often lack an explicit evidence base (Marsh and Fisher, 2005).

Professional experience about the nature of speech and language therapy is built up over many years and may constitute evidence. But there is a danger that by relying on practice wisdom and the passing of that down the generations, we do not challenge what we are doing. When we intervene in the lives of others, we should do so with the best evidence available (Johnson and Austin, 2005). This is where evidence-based practice and discussion of morals and ethics must inform practice.

Perhaps one of the reasons that these aspects of professional practice and professional identity have not been examined is because of the strong influence of the positivist paradigm in speech and language therapy. Therapy as a term derives from a medical model yet in many aspects of our work it is the social model that dominates. "Speech language pathology as a profession has fought many battles over many years to have its practice recognised as 'scientific' at the same time as internally debating the legitimacy of the scientific paradigm. The battle has left its scars in the language we use to describe what we do" (Ferguson, 2009, p.109).

The emphasis within health professions on facts and on so-called hard data (Lum, 2002) conflicts with the values-based practice espoused by many. The technical rational approach is underpinned by audit and quality standards and so has a vital role to play in the process of providing evidence for our efficacy (Fish and Coles, 1998; Anderson and van der Gaag, 2005). The delivery of care packages is described as if the packages can be designed separately from the client and administered by the clinician. This reflects a linear technocratic model requiring a front-loading of theory. The term 'professional artistry' recognises the messy uniqueness of decision making (Anderson and van der Gaag, 2005, p.3). Clinical reasoning in speech and language therapy has often been seen as a linear or logical process – this obscures the messiness and complexity of clinical reasoning in practice (Higgs et al., 2008) and under-emphasises the challenge of working in a way that truly seeks to be client-centred and build on collaborative partnership.

Non-propositional knowledge: Professional craft knowledge

> "The proliferation of types of knowing can make it unclear what rigour is left to the idea of non-propositional types of knowing. And if we are unclear what this stuff is, then the complex business of initiating new members

> into professional practice can too easily elide into mere socialisation of behaviour."
>
> (Luntley in Bondi et al., 2011, p.28)

It is this initiation into the profession that happens during the course of the speech and language therapy students' time at university. If we do not attempt to pin down the tacit knowledge, the practice wisdom used so competently by the expert practitioner, all the students are left with is the adoption of ways of behaving and models of practice that they are witness to on placement. It is our responsibility to ensure that we help the students to question some of the received wisdom that they are imbibing. We need to ensure that they are not just being exposed to a "vague sense of learning the ropes" (Luntley in Bondi et al., 2011, p.29). We need as a profession to become better at identifying and describing what makes an expert practitioner.

> "Expertise is marked, in part, by a rich capacity for attending to fine discriminations that once picked up with concepts, can become the subject matter of propositional knowledge… It is the attentional capacities, the preparedness to always see more worthy of thinking about, that marks out the distinctive contribution of expertise to many forms of professional practice."
>
> (Luntley in Bondi et al., 2011, p.40)

If we can make this expertise explicit to student practitioners they will understand the path that they need to embark on in becoming a therapist.

Brante (2010) talks of what he sees as typical of a professional situation:

> "Professionals possess knowledge of mechanisms for various phenomena but have to make delicate judgements about which ones are the optimal to use, how they should be used, and what doses are appropriate… Thus there exists – must exist if the activity is not to become routinized and in danger of being taken over by other occupations – a measure of uncertainty in a professional situation, entailing that professionals can refer to their tacit knowledge and demand discretion in conducting their work" (p.861).

The 'swampy lowlands' of professional culture, the phrase that Schön (1983) used to describe the type of subjective and context-bound knowing that practitioners need to solve problems, at times defy analysis. Exploring these lowlands is challenging for students who sometimes feel that they are in a new country without a map. In attempting to introduce it to them, we have found that the tacit knowledge base is often difficult for them to access. Crucially, the tacit knowledge has not always been scrutinised and although often referred to as practice wisdom, may have some elements that are unacceptable or unsupportable once they are more thoroughly examined. Because this tacit knowledge is largely acquired through an accumulation of experience and personal reflections by seasoned practitioners, the novice is at a disadvantage, through having no reservoir of past clinical experience on which to draw. We have been looking at ways of making this tacit knowledge more accessible, through for example asking therapists to reflect using video but have found it difficult to achieve. Clinicians are often reluctant to commit their clinical thinking to camera, and lack confidence in passing this on to students, preferring them to learn through experience, just as they did. We have wondered whether clinicians, and we include ourselves in this, find the exploration of the tacit knowledge challenging precisely because it is opaque and not easily subjected to rigorous examination. Yet we feel that the practice wisdom, the intuitive side of therapy, the 'professional artistry' (Anderson and van der Gaag, 2005) is intensely important and crucial to pass on to future practitioners. Only when we can start to describe it will it be possible to do this effectively.

According to Gustavsson (2004) in Higgs et al. (2004), "the knowledge which is shaped from long-term familiarity with an occupation (tacit knowledge) can combine with knowledge produced in research (knowledge based upon assertions) to lead development of knowledge of practical occupations" (p.44). The challenge for us as educators of speech and language therapists has been to get the balance right when introducing knowledge, both tacit and explicit, to the students.

Challenging received wisdom

Non-propositional knowledge: Clinical reasoning and the therapeutic alliance

Clinical reasoning is often seen as a separate process to the development of a therapeutic alliance whereas there is evidence that the relationship between critical thinking and interpersonal skills is linked through the key skill of empathy (Deal, 2003). In the world of psychotherapy, it is acknowledged that "the therapy relationship makes substantial and consistent contributions to patient success" (Norcross and Lambert, 2010, p.1). In speech and language therapy there has been limited exploration of the elements that make up the successful therapy relationship and we have not had discussions about the evidence behind the research into this. We have spent time exploring the actual therapy methods, measuring change on quantitative measures while ignoring the fact that "the therapy relationship accounts for why clients improve or fail to improve as much as the treatment methods used" (Norcross and Lambert, 2010, p.1). We could do well to learn from psychotherapy about how we can examine more closely the effectiveness of the therapeutic relationship.

If empathy is a central skill to establishing successful therapeutic relationships, is it one that can be taught? There is limited evidence of the effectiveness of empathy training (Erera, 1997). But we feel there should be more examination of how the skills of developing an effective therapeutic alliance are acquired. Erera (1997) describes a process where student social workers record the statements made by clients and are encouraged to consider different hypotheses to explore why the client said something, what the underlying reasons were for a statement. This deepens the student social workers' understanding of the nature of communication. They are also encouraged to examine their own statements – to explore what they meant to convey by statements they used. This kind of detailed analysis of what goes on in the development of a therapeutic relationship is not used as a method for teaching speech and language therapy students. Shouldn't we in training be encouraging much more detailed analysis of the responses we give during therapy sessions, recording the words used, and analysing these with supervisors? We don't believe that our profession has taken this approach to training speech and language therapists and this is a missing element in helping the student to understand the nature of a therapeutic relationship. It is just assumed that people either have or will develop empathy. Just because someone has empathy does not mean that they are right about the motivations and inclinations of another person; "one can be empathetic and yet misinterpret what the client means" (Erera, 1997, p.246). "Efforts to promulgate best practice or evidence-based practices without including the relationship are incomplete and potentially misleading" (Norcross and Lambert, 2010, p.1). We would welcome more examination of these aspects of the therapeutic relationship within speech and language therapy and have made a start at it in our teaching, but more evidence is required.

Teaching intervention

In preparing student practitioners for placement and then for their first job, we have been challenged by the need to teach them what intervention actually is and what has been found to be effective. The emphasis on the methods and the techniques is of course important, but without considering the whole area of the therapeutic relationship maybe we are missing the key ingredients that determine effectiveness. The student practitioner may feel that their role is to 'do something **to** the client', whereas often the emphasis should be on enabling the client to become more self-managing. The skills of the therapist in achieving this are difficult to identify and little explored.

Intervention is a relatively under-theorised and under-researched area (Martin, 2009, p.6) although this is changing with, for example, the establishment of the WhatWorks database (http://www.thecommunicationtrust.org.uk/whatworks).

But the fact remains that when the student or the practising therapist is faced with what to do with Mr X or child J on a Tuesday morning, he or she is more likely to do something within the clinical experience of the therapist, informed by possible available evidence base if it exists. Zipoli and Kennedy (2005) found that clinical experience and the opinions of colleagues were used to guide decision making more frequently than research studies or clinical practice guidelines. Wolf and Balderson (2005) found that speech-language pathologists based most of their clinical decisions on information taught during graduate programmes, clinical experience and opinions of clients. This is not because the therapist does not realise the importance of using evidence-based practice, but because there is still relatively very little available evidence for much of the routine speech and language therapy work carried out. Time is seen as a barrier for practising clinicians to access evidence. Mattingly (1998) talks about the "highly improvisational character of much clinical work, situations where the therapist suddenly 'sees' a possible story, often presented through the unexpected actions of the patient and opportunistically builds on this" (p.158). The dynamics of therapy reflect the impact of the client on the therapist, and the dynamics of individual connection, fleeting and transformational for both people involved. These are the dynamics that are hard to pin down and hard to subject to rigorous analysis. Clark in Bondi et al. (2011) makes some highly relevant points in relation to this: "Scientific evidence and knowledge are incapable of rendering the individual, improvisatory, fluid and artistic aspects of practice" (p.51), and "evidence based practice will never cover all of the issues that the individual practitioner encounters in an average day" (p.53). And in relation to social work, "if the research base is always going to be inadequate, might it be that the whole notion of basing practice on research is fundamentally flawed?" (p.50). This kind of thinking may well alarm us as a profession that has striven to make itself more credible through the use of well-structured research but it is a question that perhaps deserves more attention. There may be justification for construing therapy as necessarily experimental as long as the therapist is constantly monitoring the effects of the intervention and adapting accordingly, using such knowledge as is accessible from evidence-based practice. With the support of critical thinking and reflective practice as a crucial tool, therapy intervention can become an "open-minded search for understanding rather than the discovery of a necessary conclusion" (Kurfiss, 1989, p.42).

Non-propositional knowledge: Personal knowledge

Alongside the development of expertise of this kind, we need to support the students to contribute to the explicit and implicit standards of behaviour in the profession. "The path to expertise in any craft, discipline, profession or field is one of gradual initiation into the shared beliefs, attitudes, interests, norms and priorities that define members of that particular community of practitioners" (Vokey and Kerr in Bondi et al., 2011, p.71). We have emphasised this aspect of initiation throughout our programme.

In order to achieve this, and in the process of preparing the speech and language therapy student for the world of work, we have placed reflective practice at the centre of the curriculum. We emphasise to the students, from the beginning, the importance of reflective practice in making the clinical thinking and decision-making more explicit to ourselves. Anderson and van der Gaag (2005) talk about the importance of a reflective approach, examining personal values and beliefs and how these impact on interaction with patients (p.11). We underline to the students the importance of therapists having a self-awareness of their own values, prejudices and attitudes if they are to support change in others. Hinckley (2008) says of us as speech and language therapists: "When we compare ourselves to other related fields… we have paid much less attention to social and emotional processes within the clinical process than our counterparts" (p.x). Through reflection and skilled supervision we can probe these processes more effectively "…without critical reflection, expert practitioners run the risk of fossilization of the very patterns that defined their expertise" (Ferguson, 2008, p.vii).

We also place narrative approaches at the centre of our curriculum and have found that by introducing narrative reasoning to the students we have gained a greater understanding of the world of speech and language therapy. Storytelling is a human response to making sense of what is happening, and by using stories as a way of structuring intervention, students can be helped to see the way that narratives can shape their own identity and the professional culture that they are being introduced to. Mattingly (1998) writes about occupational therapy and reflects on her "awkward attempt to sum up an entire profession in tidy little statements, a need to get a grasp of the cultural whole" (p.ix). This is something that has challenged us in the education of students. We have used a narrative approach to help make sense of it. As we tell stories, "we create a sense of identity as clinicians. It is this identity that guides us in our clinical interactions, and intertwines with our clients' identity" (Hinckley, 2008, p.25). In the introduction to Rachel Naomi Remen's book *Kitchen Table Wisdom*, she says: "Sitting around the table telling stories is not just a way of passing time. It is the way the wisdom gets passed along" (Remen, 1996, p.xxv). It is often through hearing stories from experienced clinicians that students are introduced to the emotional and psychological aspects of clinical interactions and begin to feel that it is permissible to acknowledge doubt, and that uncertainty and recognising what works and what doesn't are key aspects of professional and personal development.

It is important for the students to be introduced to the professional identity and culture of speech and language therapy. Godsey (2011) discussed professional identity as a critical and formative process – a process, not a destination. Fagermoen (1997) studied professional identity formation in nursing and construed it as a process involving social interaction and self-reflection. Through participation in placement, professional identity is largely socially constructed. It changes over time, and develops with further and deeper exposure to a community of practice. "We may become so adapted to our professional culture that we are no longer consciously aware of how our narrative reflects the meta-narrative of the workplace and how this relates to the clients' narrative" (Hinckley, 2008, p.186). "People within a specific profession (x) will naturally tend to think like an x, see the world through the eyes of an x, notice the things that an x notices and ask the questions that an x asks about these things" (Higgs et al., 2004, p.57). The task of clinical education is to introduce and unpack these actions to the new student. But every new student brings a unique set of skills and qualities, contributing to the interaction between the student and the educator, and influencing the development of thinking of both. In running the new programme we have learned so much from the contributions of the diverse range of postgraduate students we have had, who bring with them experiences from a wide range of professions before they chose to become speech and language therapists. When faced with the traditional, monocultural aspects of our profession, the diversity of our student group has given us some important experiences as educators and we have had to face the fact that diversity may at times not be welcomed as openly as we would like to think. We have had to consider whether in a small profession, diversity may at times scare people rather than be embraced. We need to recognise the vital contribution of alternative views and perspectives brought by mature, experienced and diverse students on our programme, who of course are potential colleagues in the workplace.

As speech and language therapy has developed as a profession, a particular role has emerged for the expertise that we demonstrate. There does need to be more consideration of the fact that we may not be the only profession who works on communication and that many of the divisions between the people professions may shift during the course of the next 25 years, as it becomes clear that barriers between us may be arbitrary. We need to be alive to the possibility that we are defending our professional knowledge, which could develop more openly by interacting with other professions. We must guard against protectionism and privileging of certain skills and be prepared to draw on research from other fields on behaviour change, motivation, interaction and the role of positive psychology. It is perhaps understandable that in the early stages of the emergence of our profession we have been precious about our skills but we need to make sure that we are open to considering where our clients might benefit from the expertise of other professionals and where we can learn from other fields of practice.

So the book includes some of the stones that we have uncovered in our 'hike' so far along the combined trails of our collective careers. We are aware that in uncovering some of the stones we may unsettle ourselves and colleagues, but in the words of a Zen saying: "The most dangerous thing in the world is to think you understand something."

This book is a series of brief essays from colleagues, many of them involved in creating a new speech and language therapy programme, reflecting some of the issues we have had to confront in designing a curriculum. These essays are necessarily personal and reflective in nature, drawing on the traditions of appreciative enquiry, action research and co-production with students. Throughout the book we use 'we' to denote ourselves as speech and language therapists or clinicians – these terms are used interchangeably – and as educators of future speech and language therapists.

- Can effective and meaningful reflective practice, aimed at the development of professional knowledge, be adequately supported through the use of models of reflection which often require us to 'bend the experience to fit the tool' rather than taking personal responsibility for thinking through issues? In a period of rapid and fundamental change to the practice context, is the emphasis on purely independent and introspective reflective practice an effective approach, or is collaborative engagement with reflexive practice across and within teams, professional groups and organisations a more far-reaching strategy to effect and adapt constructively to the challenges of change? (Chapter 1)

- Why do we often provide packages of care in six weekly blocks? Is this an example of practice wisdom or poorly evidenced practice? (Chapter 2)

- Although supervision is now more widespread within the profession, does this supervision result in transformational learning for the supervisee or is the supervisory practice prevalent in the profession more about managerial accountability, managing risk and largely driven by process? (Chapter 3)

- Could therapy be conceived as a process of learning for the client, which gives them tools of self-awareness, resilience and an understanding of how to adapt in relation to the demands of their environment, in the context of their communication difficulty? How can the application of video enhance our service delivery and our support for each other? (Chapter 4)

- Why do we skirt around the spiritual aspects of speech and language therapy when these may be central to a client's self-image, particularly in responding to a traumatic event such as a stroke? (Chapter 5)

- Why is there little emphasis on learning theory in the curriculum of speech and language therapists when so much of our work should be based on an understanding of how children and adults learn? What exactly is the nature of speech and language therapy – is it a type of teaching or is it a type of rehabilitation? What are the differences between professional practice in teaching and professional practice in speech and language therapy? (Chapter 6)

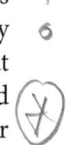

- Why, for example, are speech and language therapists in the UK mostly white women? Is this desirable or acceptable when our clients are from much more diverse social, cultural and ethnic backgrounds? (Chapters 7 and 8)

- What do we really mean by the 'service user' and what is the concept of service that we sign up for in becoming a speech and language therapist? (Chapter 9)

We have at times found the process of scrutinising our professional practices and our professional identities uncomfortable; "to reflect on the everyday taken for granted assumptions of social practices involving discourse in order to provide the opportunity for change... can be viewed as unnecessarily negative... because it will investigate ideas and practices in which ... researchers... have considerable personal, professional and potentially emotional investment" (Ferguson, 2008, p.2). We are still in the process of trying to understand just what speech and language therapy really is and while we hope to explore aspects of this in this book, we recognise that the process is an ever-changing, dynamic one.

> "The only wisdom we can hope to acquire is the wisdom of humility, humility is endless."
>
> (Eliot, 1940)

References

Anderson, C. & van der Gaag, A. (2005) *Speech and Language Therapy: Issues in Professional Practice*. London: Whurr.

Bondi, L., Carr, D., Clark, C. & Clegg, C. (2011) *Towards Professional Wisdom: Practical Deliberation in the People Professions*. Farnham: Ashgate Publishing.

Brante, T. (2010) Professional fields and truth regimes: In search of alternative approaches. *Comparative Sociology*, 9, 843–866.

Deal, K.H. (2003) The relationship between critical thinking and interpersonal skills. *The Clinical Supervisor*, 22(2), 3–19.

Eliot, T.S. (1940) Four Quartets, East Coker. http://www.davidgorman.com/4Quartets/2-coker.htm

Enderby, P. & Emerson, J. (1995) *Does Speech and Language Therapy Work?* London: Whurr.

Erera, P. (1997) Empathy training for helping professionals: Model and evaluation. *Journal of Social Work Education*, 33(2), 245–260.

Fagermoen, M.S. (1997) Professional identity: Values embedded in meaningful nursing practice. *Journal of Advanced Nursing*, 25(3), 434–441.

Ferguson, A. (2008) *Expert Practice: A Critical Discourse*. Abingdon: Plural Publishing.

Ferguson, A. (2009) The discourse of speech-language pathology. *International Journal of Speech-Language Pathology*, 11(2),.104–112.

Fish, D. & Coles, C. (1998) Professionalism eroded: Professionals under siege. In D. Fish & C. Coles (Eds) *Developing Professional Judgement in Health Care: Learning Through the Critical Appreciation of Practice*. Oxford: Butterworth-Heinemann.

Fraser, S., Lewis, V., Ding, S., Kellett, M. & Robinson, C. (2004) *Doing Research with Children and Young People*. London: Sage.

Godsey, S.R. (2011) Student perceptions of professional identity and cultural competence. Unpublished Ed.D. dissertation. Graduate School University of Minnesota.

Higgs, J. & Titchen, A. (1995) Propositional, professional and personal knowledge in clinical reasoning. In J. Higgs & M. Jones (Eds) *Clinical Reasoning in the Health Professions*. Oxford: Butterworth-Heinemann, pp.129–146.

Higgs, J., Richardson, B. and Abrandt Dahlgren, M. (2004) *Developing Practice Knowledge for Health Professionals*. London: Elsevier Health Sciences.

Hinckley, J.J. (2008) *Narrative-based Practice in Speech-Language Pathology: Stories of a Clinical Life*. Abingdon: Plural Publishing.

Johnson, M. & Austin, M.J. (2005) Evidence-based practice in the social services – implications for organizational change. calswec.berkeley.edu/files/uploads/pdf/CalSWEC/EB_0705_2.1_EBP_FinalFeb05.pdf

Kurfiss, J.G. (1989) Helping faculty foster students' critical thinking in the disciplines. In A.F. Lucas (Ed.), *New Directions for Teaching and Learning* (No. 37). San Francisco: Jossey-Bass.

Lum, C. (2002) *Scientific Thinking in Speech and Language Therapy*. Mahwah, N.J.: Lawrence Erlbaum.

Marsh, P. & Fisher, M. (2005) SCIE Report 10: Developing the evidence base for social work and social care practice. http://www.scie.org.uk/publications/reports/report10.asp

Martin, D.M. (2009) *Language Disabilities in Cultural and Linguistic Diversity*. Bristol: Multilingual Matters.

Mattingly, C. (1998) *Healing Dramas and Clinical Plots: The Narrative Structure of Experience*. Cambridge: Cambridge University Press.

Norcross J.C. & Lambert M.J. (Eds) (2010) Evidence based therapy relationships. http://www.nrepp.samhsa.gov/pdfs/Norcross_evidence-based_therapy_relationships.pdf

Remen, R.N. (1996) *Kitchen Table Wisdom: Stories That Heal*. New York: Riverhead.

Schön, D. (1983) *The Reflective Practitioner: How Professionals Think in Action*. London: Temple Smith.

Skovholt, T. & Trotter-Mathison, M. (Eds) (2011) *The Resilient Practitioner: Burnout Prevention and Self-care Strategies for Counselors, Therapists, Teachers and Healthcare Professionals*. New York: Routledge.

Wolf, T. & Balderson, J. (2005) Selection of therapy techniques for voice therapy. Poster session at the Midsouth Conference on Communication Disorders, Memphis, TN.

Zipoli, R. & Kennedy, M. (2005) Evidence-based practice among speech-language pathologists: Attitudes, utilization, and barriers. *American Journal of Speech-Language Pathology*, 14, 208–220.

1 Reflective practice in speech and language therapy

Marian McCormick

> "The term 'reflection' is now in such common use in professional education that there is considerable danger of it being taken for granted, rather than treated as problematic. Are we ceasing to be reflective about how we use 'reflection' in our discourse and in our practice? How do we practise reflection, and does it achieve what we claim it achieves?"
>
> Eraut (2004, p.47)

Reflection, problematic?

Reflection is problematic. It is problematic to define, problematic to characterise and practise in a professional context, and problematic to introduce and 'teach' to students. It is a complex concept. There is a vast literature surrounding the topic across a range of different professional groups. There are numerous definitions, published models and frameworks available to support reflective practice, derived from a variety of theoretical and epistemological orientations, which arise from different understandings of and beliefs about what can be known, and how it can be known. Epistemology is concerned with the roots of ideas, how we acquire knowledge, and how we develop concepts in our minds. Different academic disciplines, such as psychology, sociology and education, and different professions have adopted different ways of looking at the same things, and different terminology to refer to those things, which reflect their particular philosophical, intellectual, academic or professional interests.

These different understandings of reflection and reflective practice have resulted in much debate about its nature (Dewey, 1933; Kolb, 1984; Habermas,

1974; Schön 1983; Boud, Keogh and Walker, 1985; Eraut, 1994; Moon, 1999) and how it may be construed and implemented within both professional practice and educational contexts across many disciplines (Brookfield, 1995; Eraut, 1994; Jasper, 2003; Bulman and Schutz, 2004; Moon, 2004; Pollard and Anderson, 2008). There are some areas of commonality, but beyond the common there is much ongoing debate around the definition and process of reflection and the role it plays in personal, professional and academic development. The term itself has many forms: reflection, reflective practice, reflexive practice, critical reflection, reflective writing. These terms are often used interchangeably but can also be used in different and sometimes contradictory ways. As Eraut (2004) points out, the term is in such common use that it seems to have lost, rather than gained, meaning.

This chapter aims to explore the 'received wisdom' about reflective practice and how we do it, and to discuss how, as a profession, our practice of reflection could be further developed to act as a vital and innovative process for the construction of professional knowledge, and person-centred development.

Reflection is doubly problematic within speech and language therapy because 'reflective practice' has become deeply embedded within the culture of our profession, and evidence of reflective practice has become a requirement, with continued registration dependent upon it. Within speech and language therapy there is a strong professional imperative to engage in reflective practice. From the Health and Care Professions Council (HCPC):

> "(The registrant must…) understand the value of reflection on practice and the need to record the outcome of such reflection."
>
> (HCPC, 2014, p.11)

The Royal College of Speech and Language Therapists states that:

> "… critical reflective practice and continuing professional development (CPD) activities underpin and drive the maintenance of competence."
>
> (RCSLT, 2006 , p.32)

And finally, the Quality Assurance Agency:

> "The award holder should be able to: measure and evaluate critically the outcomes of professional activities; reflect on and review practice."
>
> (QAA, 2001, p.4)

Reflective practice has been deemed by all these institutions to be an essential skill in helping both students and practitioners consider their practice and link this to ongoing professional education and development, and is thus subsumed in the notion and definition of competence. We not only have to reflect, we have to show that we are reflecting.

Again this is highly problematic for us, and raises many questions, because if we don't really know and can't really define what we mean by the term, how can we practise it?

- How can we evidence or demonstrate something that we struggle to characterise?
- Are we as a profession, as suggested by Eraut (2004), unreflective and uncritical in our practice of reflection?
- Is it meaningful?
- Is it useful?
- What does it achieve in real terms?
- What is the most effective way of reflecting?
- What is 'good' reflective practice?
- What is 'good enough' reflective practice?
- If it is a requirement for ongoing registration, how is it monitored and measured?
- How will we know if we are doing it well, or well enough?

Students, especially those who have not worked within a professional context before coming onto the course and therefore have not been exposed to unconsciously accepted aspects of professional practice, invariably ask such questions. If students are being assessed on their being able to demonstrate an ability to reflect, and we as practitioners are being monitored in terms of meeting the ongoing registration requirements through our reflections on our practice and CPD activities, shouldn't we then be engaging in critical dialogue about the nature and purpose of those processes as they affect us, and the ethical and professional dilemmas that lie in the tension between professional autonomy and professional accountability? This tension arises when reflective practice is a mechanism for growth as we engage in learning and development, and simultaneously a means by which professional regulation and control can be exercised, at a variety of levels; for example, as part of academic assessments within our pre-registration programmes, in peer supervision, appraisals, and other performance management activities. We talk a lot about ethical and professional issues within our clinical context – perhaps it would be good to include in that professional discourse these broader questions relating to our professional cultures and reflection.

These questions provide a challenge to us not only as educators and those who support clinical education, but also as practitioners, to respond to and demonstrate the value and integration of reflective practice into our own professional practice. We need to come to some common understanding about the nature and purpose of reflective practice and an agreement as to how it can be used most effectively to promote practitioners to develop their work by thinking critically about their actions. As Fook, Gardner and White (2006) say, "… to interrogating [interrogate] practice in such a way that the hidden, tacit or taken for granted aspects may be properly understood and debated" (p.xii).

Such reflection on reflective practice is not just important for improving individual practice, but for developing the profession as a whole, enhancing service user experience and increasing the impact of the reflexive process on research and service development.

The context

My exploration of reflection began when I was given responsibility for enabling students on the postgraduate diploma in speech and language therapy (PGDip SLT) to learn about reflective practice in order to be able to demonstrate skills sufficient for them to meet the professional requirements for registration. Teaching reflection became a challenge central to my role as a lecturer, as it was a key area for development of student practitioners, but it also became a personal journey as I explored the nature of reflection in my own practice. When I began to teach there was little written about reflection in speech and language therapy, so I looked more widely and drew on literature from occupational therapy, teaching and nursing, where there was a wealth of information and strategies.

I started out with little confidence and a lot of PowerPoint presentations about models of reflection, and gave several lectures based on the 'received wisdom' prevalent at the time. Sadly, these initial forays into the 'teaching' of reflective practice were not successful, nor were they interesting or challenging. They resulted mainly in students expressing concern that they did not understand the topic, and demonstrating high levels of anxiety and dissatisfaction – they felt that that they did not understand what reflection was, and that they felt unprepared for the use of it during placement. This was an important learning event for me as I found myself responding primarily to the surface feedback and criticisms, instead of seeing them as symptomatic of more fundamental issues such as how adults learn, and what my role in that learning might look like. I felt a very real and uncomfortable tension about where I was and where I wanted to be, as simply lecturing about reflection, and presenting it as a 'product' had not been successful. This led me to pose questions about the nature of my knowledge about reflection, and to realise that there was significant potential to enhance both my own and my students' learning and satisfaction.

I began to explore the literature in relation to reflective practice and decided to carry out a study on the topic. There were two main aims of conducting this research project. The first was to improve my knowledge, skills and understanding in relation to the facilitation of learning about reflective practice. The second was to use that understanding to positively influence the learning of the students on the PGDip SLT. At the start of this process I was unclear even as to the questions I needed to ask, I just knew that I needed to do something better. From the point of view of quantitative research this would have been a very undesirable place to start, as without a precise and well-defined research question it is impossible to design a study to address an issue in a precise and meaningful way. However, from within a qualitative research framework, such as Action Research and grounded theory, this is not only permissible but also an acceptable initial stance, which can lead to a progressive approximation towards a set of informed and actionable outcomes. These qualitative approaches to research are concerned with real challenges within an individual's practice.

> "Action research is an enquiry conducted by the self into the self. You, a practitioner, think about your own life and work, and this involves you asking yourself why you do

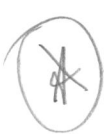

the things that you do, and why you are the way that you are. When you produce your research report, it shows how you have carried out a systematic investigation into your own behaviour, and the reasons for that behaviour. The report shows the process you have gone through in order to achieve a better understanding of yourself, so that you can continue developing yourself and your work."

(McNiff, 2002, p.6)

The Action Research process, in common with grounded theory approaches, has as a central feature a cyclical process involving 'cycles of learning and change', which provided a realistic structure within which I could, over time and with experience, refine my ideas and identify the strategies which were most effective in achieving my overall goal of facilitating reflective practice. Through talking with and listening to the students over a 5-year period, I began to notice certain patterns and issues, and year on year could compare the outcomes, and look for similarities and differences in what worked, how students responded to new ideas and how they began to respond to and develop their reflective practice. Through this process I came to a deeper understanding and clearer development of my ideas about what reflection was and what it was not. I also saw that reflecting on and examining my own work, raising questions as to how effective I was being, and generating ideas as to how I could do it better, was research-minded, and I was engaging in a form of 'practitioner-led' research.

"A defining condition of being human is that we have to understand the meaning of our experience. For some, any uncritically assimilated explanation by an authority figure will suffice. But in contemporary societies we must learn to make our own interpretations rather than act on the purposes, beliefs, judgements and feelings of others. Facilitating such understanding is the cardinal goal of adult education. Transformative learning develops autonomous thinking."

(Mezirow, 1997, p.5)

The process of carrying out this study over such a period of time has become a story within a story. The larger narrative involves the development of my knowledge and understanding of theories, ideas and how to think about and present reflective practice. The smaller narrative is dependent on the first, but has a much more personal and integrative function: a change in my personal and professional practice and the value I place on reflective practice, which now has a fundamental impact on my teaching.

Received wisdom

Received wisdom tells us that reflective practice is primarily about learning from experience. It is often portrayed as an individual, introspective and retrospective activity, usually achieved through the use of (in a professional capacity) a model or framework of reflection, which has, as a product of that activity, a piece of reflective writing, a demonstration of the learning that has taken place.

Reflective practice as an individual activity

Reflective practice is essentially an individual activity. It involves each of us in generating and selecting the topic of our reflections, and in engaging with the content in describing the experience, reflecting on it and learning from the experience, based on our own responses to and understanding of our experiences (Boud et al., 1985; Mezirow, 1981; Fook et al., 2006).

Individual attitudes towards reflective practice can vary on a continuum from 'navel-gazing' – an unnecessary or redundant activity and the first thing that can be dropped in the context of ever-increasing professional demands – through to being perceived as self-indulgence, or to being viewed and valued as a necessary and vital tool for personal and professional development. The value we give to something has an impact on how we prioritise it. If we see a purpose to something, we tend to value it more highly; this holds true whether we are talking about ourselves as individuals or of the organisations in which we work. Closely allied to the individual aspect of reflective practice, and the personal values that drive our engagement with it, is the concept of intentionality – there is a big difference between being required or told to do something, and of seeing the inherent value and benefit of an activity in which we then intentionally take part.

> "One of the biggest difficulties, when other people are in control of our learning, is that we cannot then own it. As a result we see other people as being responsible for it. Ownership of learning is fundamental to the principles of lifelong learning."
>
> (Hinchliff, 1999, p.68)

The thing that sets reflection in our professional lives apart from everyday reflection is intentionality; as Eyler, Giles and Schmiede (1996) note, reflection "need not be a difficult process but it does need to be a purposeful and strategic process" (p.16).

Reflective practice as product or process?

There is no single correct way to reflect, neither is there one single best way to represent the outcome of such reflection, but through working with students in supporting the development of their reflective practice, a number of things have emerged as being significant enablers to this development. From a pedagogical perspective, the most significant outcome has been the recognition that effective engagement with reflective practice is a developmental process, and that presenting it as a continuum of development can help students to see it as a process rather than focusing on producing a 'product'. They begin to see themselves move from simple description of concrete experiences to engaging in reflective practice that involves more abstract, meta-cognitive strategies, resulting in changes in both the nature and content of their reflections. Their focus moves from having to produce a piece of work to active engagement in the process of learning, recognising patterns of behaviour and underlying assumptions and motivations. Students appear more willing to ask questions; to use trial and error to weigh up alternative courses of action; to make mistakes and feel able to acknowledge them; and to be able to talk about where they are and where they have come from in terms of reflective skills. This element of self-assessment and an ability to identify and work with personal strengths and vulnerabilities has had a growing acknowledgement within the assessment strategy literature, and shares important themes with the recent values-based initiatives within healthcare.

Excerpt from student work

> "New information is only a resource in the adult learning process" (Mezirow 1997, p.10). In other words, adults use the knowledge given to them as a foundation to build and expand upon for themselves. This type of learning is not about achieving a final goal, but is, instead, an ever-evolving process of revealing information to foster new ideas, theories and discoveries. Once the adult student accepts the responsibility for her own learning, she becomes independent of the teacher and no longer just accepts what is being told as correct, but rather seeks her own answers to any questions. I started this course determined that I would graduate with distinction. I have since decided that that is no longer the end goal for me. It is more important to me to complete this course feeling confident in my practice as a speech and language therapist and inspired to continue to learn throughout my career. Whether I graduate with distinction or not, my learning does not end."

Excerpt from student work

> " 'Reflection' as an idea was difficult to understand to begin with, due to my perception of a lack of structure and so I did not understand what was expected of me. Therefore I was not able to create a plan-of-action. I however recognised, through reassurance, that it was okay not to understand at that point in time; that "becoming is better than being" (Dweck, 2006, p.25); I needed to trust the process. I learnt to associate success with the learning process over time, not just the end goal."

Speech and Language Therapy and Professional Identity

Excerpt from student work

> "I recognise that I am only at the beginning of my learning journey, with regards to challenging my assumptions and values about success, but consider this a positive step to developing myself as a practitioner. I have become aware of my fixed mindset and the limitations this might pose on my practice, in terms of limiting my effectiveness and creativity, as well as recognising the demanding rules I impose upon myself, which bolster this fixed mindset... Central to this process of change, is regular critical reflection, enabling me to understand my own values, attitudes and beliefs, and work with them in a constructive manner."

Such an approach can promote increasing acceptance and willingness to engage with the complex, the incomplete, and the unanswerable issues which are increasingly part of professional practice in the current social, economic and political climate. At some stages of development the use of a structured, model-based approach may be helpful in building confidence, but it is incumbent on us as facilitators of this process to make clear that this may be viewed as a stage in the development of reflective practice, and that there is a lot more that may be experienced as reliance on external structure diminishes and the contextual dialogue with self begins to flourish. "Reflective practice skills are acquired and developed gradually through practice and over time, rather than in any one course or package" (Bulman and Schutz, 2004, p.27).

Finding ways to support students to be able to articulate their learning to demonstrate their engagement, broaden their perspectives, establish and understand their personal frameworks for practice, and also provide a basis for the generalisation of their personal reflections into the wider context of self in society has been the goal. In the extracts above the sense of movement, process and individual responsibility for learning emerge as central themes of the students' understanding and engagement with reflective practice.

Reflective practice as an introspective activity

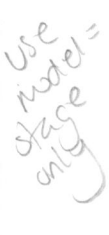

Why we reflect can range from the functional goal of meeting our professional requirements to wanting to engage critically with issues within our work contexts, identifying potential areas for change within our services and practice environments, and with a real desire to develop our professional knowledge, skills and understanding.

Reflective practice had its origins in radical roots, deeply linked to the ideas central to professionalism of taking responsibility for and responding to the context of one's practice in an autonomous and accountable manner. It involved self-assessment and the questioning and appraisal of the social, political and organisational structures in which practice was situated and the process of articulating and engaging in the discourse of change. The context in which reflective practice is often situated within the professional sphere has altered, and a distinction has arisen between what could be construed as the transactional and the transformative aspects of the concept.

The **transactional face** of reflective practice is that which conforms to the requirement to reflect, and sees reflection as a product; a routine activity that, while meeting minimal requirements, is often cursory, procedural, superficial, and functional; a safe recording of experience as it relates to meeting externally imposed targets, which does not carry any potential for criticism. In both professional and academic contexts, such an approach can lead to reflective practice becoming "another technology of professional surveillance, or reduce it to a set of learning outcome indicators or learning objectives" (Fook et al., 2006, p.xiii).

The **transformative face** of reflective practice presents an alternative approach; a process rather than a product, one which has the potential to encourage and develop self-awareness, self-management and self-assessment, all of which are central to the development of autonomous and effective practice, and key to advancing clinical knowledge, skills and understanding. "Critical reflection is not an innocent practice; it has transformative potential. By offering the chance to reflect, rethink and re-experience our professional lives as a struggle over competing values, practices and social relations, it goes beyond 'benign introspection'" (Woolgar, 1988, p.22, in Fook et al., 2006, p.xiii).

True reflective practice requires us to identify and acknowledge the frequently unexamined assumptions and values that we each carry with us, which shape our response to, and functioning within, the professional context. It also requires us to engage with what Egan (2008, p.52) calls 'the pragmatics of values' in which he clearly states that values are not ideals, they are a set of practical criteria each of us have for making decisions and as such they are drivers of our behaviour. "Working values help (therapists) make decisions on how to proceed. Therefore reviewing the values that drive your behaviours … is not optional."

Reflection gives us an opportunity to explore our core values, and provides a way for us to work out how to improve our practice in a way that has meaningful application, and that brings the multiple demands and clinical complexities of our work into the open. It can provide a means to explore issues of challenge and stress, personal growth and development; difficult issues such as handling interpersonal conflict, and an avenue to receive affirmation and encouragement.

Excerpt from student work

"I had always felt confident in my ability to try to see things from other perspectives; however, this feeling was soon shattered during the first lecture of this module. When presented with the statement below by Beckett and Maynard, everything I had ever considered about myself as being an open minded, free thinking, unbiased individual, who is able to give balanced views on matters, was promptly blown away... 'Although we are all unique, the values we hold are much less individual than we would perhaps like to think. They are shaped in large part by the society around us and by the particular subsection of society in which we find ourselves: our age group, our gender, our ethical community, our geographical community, our social class and so on. We do not notice this all the time, because we tend to assume that the values we share with those around us are just common sense. It is really only when we compare the kinds of assumptions we make now with those made at other times, or that are made in other places, or sections of society, that we realise that many of the values we take for granted are not inevitable, but are the result of a particular local consensus.'"

(Beckett and Maynard, 2013, pp.14–15)

Excerpt from student work

"Before beginning the course I assumed everyone would be quite similar, but I could not be more wrong. Inevitably students are all similar in that they are drawn to a career in speech and language therapy, which demands certain personality characteristics and other specific qualities. However, there are so many other aspects that differ – life experiences, previous study, jobs, age, priorities and values, preferred client groups, pathways to this point in time. This means that each student will become a completely different therapist; no two therapists will be the same. This is an encouraging yet disconcerting thought, as the ability to transform from student to therapist largely rests on understanding who we are, our values, attitudes and beliefs – it will be an ongoing individual and personal journey."

Excerpt from student work

"At the start of this course I didn't believe that reflection was part of my inherent value system. I struggled to see how I would be able to apply something I didn't believe was valid (Mezirow, 1997). As the course progressed it became obvious that of course reflection was part of my belief system, the use of Gibbs' reflective tool (1988) has helped me to formalise this process. I had been searching for a concrete answer to what reflection was, but what I actually needed to do was embark on negotiation of my embedded values of 'subconscious' reflection and use it in a different way. I feel I have undergone some transformation from a subconscious reflector to a more active reflector. Now I understand this I can dynamically use reflection to challenge my inherent and preconceived ideas and values."

(Abrahamsson, 1981, cited in Usher, 1985)

Although reflection is an individual and introspective process it is not enough just to say we do it; we have to provide some evidence that reflection, and learning, has taken place. Reflection is not directly observable, nor easily described, yet ultimately it has an audience to whom the results and impact of that reflection need to be represented and communicated. The challenge is how might that representation of learning be best demonstrated within both the academic and professional contexts?

Beyond the individual and the introspective

Reflection is therefore both individual and introspective in nature: what we believe about it is fundamental in shaping and influencing both our willingness to engage with the practice and our level of engagement. The challenge to the received wisdom is not to the individual nature of the practice per se, but to the belief that that is all it is. Reflective practice occurs within a **context** which both influences and shapes our experience of it, and provides an opportunity for us to influence and shape it. Reflective practice involves **discomfort** as we come across new information and experience challenges to our previously unexamined assumptions, behaviours and beliefs. It also invites **collaboration**.

The context of reflective practice

All learning, and all reflective practice, occurs within a context, and that context is powerful in shaping and either constraining or liberating each of us to engage with our immediate environment and the larger, societal and political forces that determine the context in which that occurs. Bronfenbrenner (1994) argues that "in order to understand human development, one must consider the entire ecological system in which growth occurs" (p.1643). His ecological models of development describe five subsystems which interact to provide the context for individual growth and development throughout the human lifespan, and is one of the most widely-known examples of systems thinking. Systems thinking as a discipline seeks to examine and describe the dynamic interactions, patterns of influence and complex interrelationships that exist between an individual, and the social, cultural, organisational and institutional contexts in which they live and grow. Key to Bronfenbrenner's model is the concept of the bi-directional impact of environment on people, and of people on environment – and the individual's role in changing and influencing their context. We can be influenced and inspired by those around us and the ethos of the networks and relationships with which we engage, or our sense of agency and voice can be undermined by those same social, cultural and environmental factors.

The challenge of such models to the received wisdom about reflective practice is that individual practice takes place within, and has the potential for impact upon, spheres of influence beyond the personal and the introspective. Thus those within the profession who take responsibility for the leadership of others – managers, supervisors, placement educators, and academics – must take responsibility for the context that they create and the impact of their actions and decisions on the facilitation of these key professional skills. This underlying professional culture is the context in which professional decision-making and ethical practice is embedded; it plays not only a powerful role in establishing the value of different aspects of professional practice, it also determines and defines the purpose and parameters of that practice, in terms of what is prioritised, and how certain activities are supported, e.g., reflective practice. If we see a purpose to something, we tend to value it more highly. Such choices determine and exhibit the genuine ethos of an organisation, institution or profession, as they prescribe the actions or behaviours which will be rewarded or censured.

> "Practice in health and welfare takes place in the context of powerful organizational and professional cultures. Yet, the concept of culture is often taken for granted and its capacity to shape what can be thought, said or done is ignored. [...] cultures are locally accomplished and reproduced and can sustain the tacit practices of occupations, organizations and teams, and indeed may be used to resist the sorts of approaches to policy and practice change usually associated with rational approaches to governance."
>
> (Fook et al., 2006, p.22)

The implications of this thinking on reflective practice are that if we consider only the individual and introspective dimensions of reflective activity, we diminish the impact of the process on the individual's ability to go beyond the immediate perspective, and to explore the wider implications for the transformation of practice. "The focus of critical reflection is therefore the transformation of the way that practitioners view the world and their place in it... The outcome of this process is changed conceptual perspectives" (Carr and Kemmis, 1986).

Reflective practice might then be considered in relation to two themes or dimensions; our individual identity and our professional role. Pollard and Anderson (2008) identify as central to the discussion of reflection in teaching, "a key issue is [that of] their identities as unique individuals and how they relate these identities to the roles that they must fulfil" (p.115). An example of this from within our own professional community is the continuing divide between those who do research and those who don't, and although we acknowledge at one level the need for us all to engage with and contribute to the research process and the evidence base for what we do, that divide remains. At the centre of this divide is the relationship between knowledge and practice, and whether we see ourselves as predominantly consumers of knowledge, reading and applying the research produced by others, or as producers and contributors to the knowledge base of the profession. How we see ourselves, our professional identity, and our role, will determine to a large extent the degree of comfort we have in being willing to engage in new spheres or arenas of practice, and adopt what Rolfe, Jasper and Freshwater (2010, p.32) call "a full professional role as practitioners, educationalists and researchers".

Our daily practice experiences can become a form of information-generating activity. Turning information into knowledge is an active process and critical reflection is a key way of doing it. Through the process of noticing what we are doing, articulating our choices and raising questions arising from our clinical experiences, we can look at generated theories and see whether or not our practice experience confirms, adds to, or challenges research generated by others. Action Research as a research model is just that: a series of iterative cycles of action and reflection arising out of the lived experience of a practitioner. Rolfe et al. (2010, p.13) states that reflection "enables practitioners to begin to build their own personal and situational knowledge and theory base so that they are able to respond not only from their scientific knowledge, but also from their experiential knowledge".

Discomfort and dissonance

Professional practice is not always easily defined or managed; parts of it can be disturbing and challenging, complex and messy. The role of leaders, managers and educators within the profession should encompass the broaching of these uncomfortable truths, and the demonstration of means and strategies by which students and qualified practitioners can be supported to address the myriad demands, paradoxes and inconsistencies they will face.

Integral to this process is the experience of 'cognitive dissonance' (Festinger, 1957); the psychological discomfort one feels when confronted with new information or ideas that conflict with those already held, or familiar. This discomfort can act as a catalyst for development by motivating us to reduce the 'dissonance' through resolving the inconsistency between the new ideas and experiences and those previously held, by working through the issues and restoring internal consistency. However, another response to the experience of cognitive dissonance is to avoid the psychological stress by avoiding situations and information that are likely to increase it, retreating into our previously-held ideas and into familiar territory, and seeking support from others who share the same beliefs, again restoring internal consistency through rejection of the uncomfortable alternatives.

Cognitive dissonance is an important construct in both personal and professional growth, and particularly in relation to embracing and engaging in change. Other influential writers, such as Mezirow (1995) and Dweck (2000), refer to transformation of 'frames of reference' and the 'growth mind-set', and the anxiety that can often be experienced by individuals as they engage with significant learning. It is crucial to recognise the challenge this presents both to students, and to practitioners who are developing and extending the remit of their personal practice and the framework and assumptions that sustain habitual patterns of action. Discomfort and challenge are unsettling and therefore, at one level, worth avoiding – reflection then must form a larger part of both the educative and professional development process. "Regardless of their magnitude and importance, choices present themselves to us constantly, and critical reflection offers a method for helping us to think and act in a mindful, considered and systematic way in order to make the crucial decisions that practice demands" (Rolfe et al., 2011, p.13).

Excerpts from student work

> "I am aware that cognitive dissonance will persist and manifest itself in various forms along my learning journey and yet I recognise that confronting it is a process which allows for the greater development of critical self-reflection, professional identity and overall increased competence."

> "It has not been in any way an easy process, but through time and being open to new knowledge and environments

on this course, I can use this experience to help me empathise with clients experiencing similar uncertainty and change in their world or seeing things from a different perspective. Having experienced anxiety and a reluctance to change my thinking, I can empathise with those who are experiencing panic and initial resistance to the new situation in which they find themselves. My relatively 'safe' experience of uncertainty will also assist me when it occurs in practice. Life, as we know, is never certain and is always changing. By learning to deal with uncertainty, fear of the unknown, anxiety of change and their challenges, in this positive learning environment, I feel better equipped with new tools to add to my box that I can use with future clients and family/carers."

There are implications for how we can support and encourage students, and each other, to engage in the discomfort and challenge, and to view them as an essential and desirable part of both personal, intellectual and professional development. This can be achieved in part through how the role of reflection is presented and embedded in our professional culture, but also in acknowledging that intellectual and emotional dissonance are catalysts for change. This can be supported via small group interaction and dialogue, where the impact of new ideas and the collaborative discussions and sharing of knowledge and resources can both allow and promote exploration of new ideas to be assimilated and accommodated into existing schema.

"Introspection is the dominant mode of reflective practice… it is a predominantly individualistic and personal exercise (Reynolds & Vince 2004) in which practitioners tend to focus on their own thoughts, feelings, behaviours and evaluations… the onus stays on the individual to reflect upon and evaluate their own practice… What is lacking is any mutual, reciprocal, shared process."

(Finlay, 2006, p.7)

Collaboration: Sharing and widening the impact of reflective practice

Another challenge to received wisdom is that reflection on our practice should be exclusively an individual activity. Finlay (2006, p.12) makes the point that one danger of reflection remaining solely in the individual domain is that "All too often the process may simply rationalise existing practice". When we systematically and intentionally reflect on our practice we create an opportunity to reach out to others who are working in a similar way with similar intent, who are also generating questions and seeking ways of exploring new approaches to similar issues. The difference between simply rationalising existing practice, and affirming it in collaboration with others in a wider context is significant; if we only ever pose questions to ourselves, we will always only get our own perspective back. Feedback and questioning from others provide a wider perspective, opportunities for effective partnerships and collaboration, and the construction of professional knowledge. McNiff (2002, p.2) talks of "the power of sharing ideas to generate new ones". Critical reflection can increase our sense of professional and personal agency in identifying and working towards positive change. A natural extension of this concept for those who have their reflective practice supported in this way, is the generalisation of personal reflections into the wider context of self in society and the use of these to engage in a dialogue with others to promote wider change and understanding. What we understand reflective practice to be will be formative in how we use it in a professional context to encourage and incorporate it into our professional structures for encouraging and supporting ongoing professional development.

Reflective practice and models of reflection

> "No type of reflection is better than another; each has its own value for different purposes."
>
> (Taylor, 2006, p.103)

> "There is no single correct way to do reflective writing. There are in fact many styles and techniques that people use to help them get the most out of their learning experiences…"
>
> (RCSLT, 2007)

The use of a model or framework of reflection is a very common strategy for supporting reflective practice. Received wisdom seems to imply that it doesn't really matter which model you use as long as you choose one that 'works best' for you. This raises several questions: On which basis does one choose? And if it doesn't matter which one, does this suggest that they are all the same, and as good as each other? Models of reflection derive from a variety of theoretical and epistemological frameworks; this means that each will be constructed around the beliefs, assumptions and priorities of the discipline with which the author identifies. These underpinnings determine whether a model is prescriptive or vague, categorical or dimensional, and also the degree to which it promotes broad social discourse or emphasises personal introspection. It is therefore important to consider the assumptions and orientations that underlie different models and frameworks, as these influence both what can be explored in reflective practice, and how it is explored. The theoretical position adopted by a model or framework for reflection will profoundly influence the perspectives taken for, as stated by Raddon (2010), the philosophical stance, informs the methodology and provides context for its logic and criteria; it also links the choice of methods to the desired outcomes, and determines the techniques or procedures employed to explore a topic.

Reflection, if introduced only from the perspective of requiring the use of a model of reflection, runs the risk of becoming little more than an elaborate essay plan or a recipe which when followed results in a perfectly formed exemplar: the ingredients are selected and combined in a certain way, and processed according to a prescribed sequence. At some stages of development students can find such a structured approach helpful and facilitative in building initial skills and confidence. However, it is incumbent on us educators and practitioners, as facilitators of this process, to make clear that this may be viewed as a stage in the development of both learning and reflective practice, and that there is a lot more that may be experienced as reliance on external structure diminishes and the dialogue with self, and others, begins to flourish.

Excerpts from student work

> "Since reflection is something completely new to me, I will find it most beneficial to write and reflect freely, unrestricted to a reflection model. The models can be viewed as tools that limit and hinder honest, truthful,

effective reflection. This reflective log will be approached in the same way professionals often take a case history: by allowing the client to tell his/her story, leading to more detailed information. Therefore I will avoid answering a series of limiting questions via a framework, and instead reflect freely to yield a more effective and holistic reflection."

"Through reflection I'm becoming more attuned to examining the way I approach my work and this process should help me to continually develop my practice. I've accepted that my values, attitudes, beliefs and emotional experiences influence my cognitive process, and potentially my therapeutic interactions, and that I need to be conscious of this."

Reflection as a retrospective activity

Many models and frameworks used to support reflection adopt a retrospective stance – the incident or precipitating event is reviewed and analysed from a position that is chronologically removed, so that distance is created which allows the experience to be described, analysed and exposed to alternative perspectives and ideas which help to reframe or extend learning. These are valuable and necessary elements of reflective practice. The challenge to the received wisdom is that in order to have an impact, the outcomes of reflection need to also have a future orientation; a recognition of the learning that has taken place; and the implications for change and development, both at a personal and at a professional level.

Excerpts from student work

"What I have learned about myself in the last few months is that I often see things and analyse them but fail to make changes. I can even go as far as making a plan but fail at its implementation. After familiarising myself with the factors that might influence my resistance to change and barriers to learning, I feel better equipped and have started making some changes by setting small and realistic goals. This essay is supporting me on my journey to change. Through writing it, I keep discovering new things and this is the start of the process of becoming a competent reflective practitioner."

"My learning on this module has been characterised by my realisation of the significance of autonomy as a key skill, both as an adult learner and in order to become an effective practitioner. I have grown in autonomy in the sense that I am far less influenced by others when making decisions and importance life choices… However, the challenge I am faced with now is to resist the tendency to receive knowledge as an 'empty vessel', but instead to continuously question the purpose of my learning so that I can direct it in a way that will help me achieve my long term goals."

"Through reflection I can see which areas I need to work on for the future, and I am now aware that reflection is most valuable when it becomes reflexive, by learning from experiences and reacting to what I have learnt I am able to bring about change whether that is at an individual or a structural level."

Conclusion

This chapter aimed to explore the 'received wisdom' about reflective practice, and to discuss how, as a profession, our practice of reflection could be developed to act as a vital and innovative process for the construction of professional knowledge. We are working in an ever-changing and complex professional arena, and our personal journeys are happening in the context of a much wider political and social context where restructuring, economic policies, and many forces outside of our sphere of influence shape the environment in which we practice, and how we practice.

There are many barriers we experience in reflection and it is important to recognise that "circumstances conducive to reflection need to be created" (Boud, 2010, p.34), and this is a responsibility that we all share, personally, professionally and organisationally. Wherever we work, and whatever our role in our community of speech and language therapy practice, there will be challenges in addressing the fundamental question of the role we want reflective practice to play in the culture of our profession.

This exploration of reflection within the speech and language therapy context started out as a solitary journey with the specific aim of teaching a 'product' and has ended up, as most journeys do, far from its original destination, and has become a collaborative and joint process with both colleagues and students. What we have learned is that reflective practice cannot be comfortably reduced to a set of models and useful techniques which can be acquired, mastered and applied. The hope of this chapter is to suggest that the power of reflective practice is in its open-endedness, and its essential developmental nature. It also suggests that the 'why' and the 'how' of reflection go far beyond techniques, frameworks and models, which, if not approached critically, can result in a reductionist and domesticating process rather than a creative and dynamic orientation to learning and personal and professional development characterised by a willingness and an intent to explore assumptions, and to question and to discover, through genuine curiosity. It acknowledges the context in which practice is situated and challenges us to seek ways in which to work collaboratively within and across teams.

Reflection is ultimately about learning, and making meaning. It involves a purposeful, deliberate and intentional approach to our practice and professional development, incorporating and acknowledging both the cognitive and affective domains of our learning; the ipsative and developmental nature of the process and an ability to articulate the impact of that process on our own practice and the wider systems in which our practice is situated. The implications for individuals and for the profession might be to consider ways in which we could work towards incorporating such an approach into the professional culture, as a means of monitoring engagement with standards of reflective practice, and encouraging practitioners to construct professional narratives; showing how they have understood and applied the principles of professional development in their own particular context; and writing about the impact of new ideas, approaches, collaborations and partnerships on the enhancement and extension of their knowledge, skills and understanding. I propose this because, along the way, my experience of reflective practice has been "*...a far juicier, fraught and exhilarating process than might have been* concluded from instructional manuals setting out objectives, strategies, [and] competencies" (Willis, 2000, p.62).

In a period of rapid and fundamental change to the practice context it is important to ask:

- Is the emphasis on purely independent and individualised reflective practice an effective way of understanding and using reflective activities?

- Could collaborative engagement with reflexive practice across professional groups within teams and institutions become a more far-reaching strategy to effect and adapt constructively to the challenges of change?

- How best can we work together to ensure that in our professional culture we are working towards adopting and supporting practices, at the personal, educational and managerial and institutional levels, that are effective in promoting the development of individuals and of the profession?

"...there ain't no journey what don't change you some."

(David Mitchell, 2004, *Cloud Atlas*)

References

Ash, S.L. & Clayton, P.H. (2009) Generating, deepening, and documenting learning: The power of critical reflection in applied learning. *Journal of Applied Learning in Higher Education,* 1, 25–48.

Beckett, C. & Maynard, A. (2013) *Values and Ethics in Social Work*. London: Sage Publications.

Boud, D. and Associates (2010) *Assessment 2020: Seven Propositions for Assessment Reform in Higher Education*. Sydney: Australian Learning and Teaching Council.

Boud, D. & Walker, D. (1998) *Promoting reflection in professional courses: The challenge of context*, Studies in Higher Education, 23(2), pp.191-206.

Boud, D., Keogh, R. and Walker, D. (1985) *Reflection, Turning Experience into Learning*. Abingdon: Routledge.

Bronfenbrenner, U. (1994) Ecological models of human development. *International Encyclopedia of Education*, Vol 3, 2nd ed. Oxford: Elsevier.

Brookfield, S.D. (1995) *Becoming a Critically Reflective Teacher*. San Francisco: Jossey-Bass.

Bulman, C. & Schutz, S. (2004) (Eds) *Reflective Practice in Nursing: The Growth of the Professional Practitioner*, 3rd ed. Oxford: Blackwell Scientific Publications.

Carr, W. & Kemmis, S. (1986). *Becoming Critical: Knowing Through Action Research*. Geelong: Deakin University Press.

Dewey, J. (1933) *How We Think. A Restatement of the Relation of Reflective Thinking to the Educative Process*, Revised ed. Boston: D.C.Heath.

Dweck, C.S. (2000). *Self-Theories: Their Role in Motivation, Personality, and Development*. Philadelphia: Psychology Press.

Dweck, C.S. (2006). *Mindset*. New York: Random House.

Egan, G. (2007) *The Skilled Helper: A Problem-Management and Opportunity Development Approach to Helping*. USA: Thomson Brooks/Cole.

Eraut, M. (1994) *Developing Professional Knowledge and Competence*. London: Falmer.

Eraut, M. (2000) Non-formal learning and tacit knowledge in professional work. *British Journal of Educational Psychology*, 70, 113–136.

Eraut, M. (2004) The practice of reflection. *Learning in Health and Social Care*, 3(2), 47–52.

Eyler, J., Giles, D.E. & Schmiede, A. (1996) A practitioner's guide to reflection in service-learning. In S.L. Ash & P.H. Clayton (2009) *Journal of Applied Learning in Higher Education*, 1, Fall 2009, 25–48.

Festinger, L. (1957) *A Theory of Cognitive Dissonance*. California: Stanford University Press.

Finlay, L. (2008) Reflecting on 'reflective practice'. PBPL Paper 52. A discussion paper prepared for PBPL CETL; www.open.ac.uk/pbpl.

Fook, J., Gardner, F. & White, S. (2006) *Critical Reflection in Health and Social Care*. Maidenhead: Open University Press.

Gibbs, G. (1988) *Learning by Doing: A Guide to Teaching and Learning Methods*. Oxford: Further Education Unit, Oxford Polytechnic.

Giroux, H.A. (2011) *On Critical Pedagogy*. London: Continuum.

Habermas, J. (1974) *Theory and Practice*. London: Heinemann.

Health and Care Professions Council (HCPC) (2014) HPC Standards of Proficiency – Speech and Language Therapists; www.hcpc-uk.org.uk.

Hinchliff, S. (1999) *The Practitioner as Teacher*. Oxford: Baillière Tindall.

Jasper, M. (2003) *Beginning Reflective Practice* (Foundations in Nursing and Health Care). Cheltenham: Thomas Nelson.

Kolb, D.A. (1984) *Experiential Learning: Experience as the Source of Learning and Development.* Englewood Cliffs, NJ: Prentice Hall.

Larrivee, B. (2000) Transforming teaching practice: Becoming the critically reflective teacher. *Reflective Practice*, 1(3), 293–307.

McNiff, J. (2002) Action research for professional development; Concise advice for new action researchers. http://www.jeanmcniff.com/ar-booklet.asp

Mezirow, J. (1997) Transformative learning: Theory to practice. *New Directions for Adult and Continuing Education*, 74, 5–12.

Mezirow, J. (1981) A critical theory of adult learning and education. *Adult Education Quarterly*, 32(3), 3–24.

Mitchell, D. (2004) *Cloud Atlas.* London: Hodder & Stoughton.

Moon, J. (1999) *Reflection in Learning and Professional Development.* London: Kogan Page.

Moon, J. (2004) *A Handbook of Reflective and Experiential Learning.* London: Routledge Falmer.

Pollard, A. & Anderson, J. (2008) *Reflective Teaching: Evidence-informed Professional Practice*, 3rd ed. London: Continuum.

Quality Assurance Agency subject benchmarks, speech and language therapy (2001). http://www.qaa.ac.uk/en/Publications/Documents/Subject-benchmark-statement-Health-care-programmes---Speech-and-Language-Therapy.pdf

Raddon, A. (2010) http://www2.le.ac.uk/colleges/socsci/documents/research-training-presentations/EpistFeb10.pdf

Rolfe, G., Jasper, M. and Freshwater, D. (2010) *Critical Reflection in Practice: Generating Knowledge for Care*, 2nd ed. Basingstoke: Palgrave Macmillan.

RCSLT (2006) *Communicating Quality* 3, p.32.

RCSLT (2007) Powerpoint presentation on reflective practice online www.rcslt.org.uk.

Schön, D. (1983) *The Reflective Practitioner: How Professionals Think in Action.* New York: Basic Books.

Taylor, B.J. (2006) *Reflective Practice: A Guide for Nurses and Midwives.* Sydney: Allen & Unwin.

Usher, R. (1985) Beyond the anecdotal: Adult learning and the use of experience. *Studies in the Education of Adults*, 17(1), 59–74.

Willis, P. (2000) Expressive and arts-based research: Presenting lived experience in qualitative research. In P. Willis, E. Smith and E. Collins (Eds) *Being, Seeking, Telling: Expressive Approaches to Qualitative Adult Education Research.* Flaxton, Queensland: Post Pressed, pp.35–64.

Woolgar, S. (Ed.) (1988) *Knowledge and Reflexivity.* London: Sage Publications.

2 To intervene or not to intervene

An exploration of the conflicts and dilemmas for the paediatric speech and language therapist in practice

Aoife Gallagher

> "Quality of professional practice will be achieved and improved on primarily by individual professionals working with integrity in a critically reflective way."
> (RCSLT, 2006, p.31)

The Royal College of Speech and Language Therapists (RCSLT) states that the speech and language therapist's scope of practice is "to provide evidence-based services that anticipate and respond to the needs of individuals who experience speech, language, communication or swallowing difficulties" through the engagement of clients and families and to "reduce the impact of these difficulties on people's wellbeing and their ability to participate in daily life" (RCSLT, 2006, p.2). The American Speech and Hearing Association (ASHA) provides four guiding principles for speech and language therapy services for young children, which need to be: (a) family-centred and culturally and linguistically responsive; (b) promote children's ability to participate, (c) be coordinated and collaborative; and (d) be driven by or based on the highest quality evidence available (ASHA 2008a, b, c, d). Speech Pathology Australia (SPA) also sets out clearly that evidence-based practice, functional outcomes for clients, responsiveness to the individual needs of the client and family and collaborative working are central to the speech language pathologist's role (SPA, 2010). There is consensus therefore about what constitutes the core values which should underpin the practice of paediatric speech and language therapists and which should guide paediatric speech and language therapy models of service delivery. These are: (a) the use of the highest quality research evidence available, underpinning our decision making in order to achieve the best outcomes; (b) responsiveness to the individual needs of the client and family; (c) partnership with the families and clients we serve; and (d) outcomes which have an impact on the client's ability to participate in the community. This chapter explores the practice of using prescribed models of intervention in paediatric speech and language therapy service delivery in the context of the values outlined above. In terms of evidence-based practice, it reviews some of the most recent intervention studies in relation to dosage. It explores the issue of prescribed models of intervention in terms of working in partnership with our clients and families. It highlights the importance of critically evaluating the application of untested intervention levels in order to best serve the needs of children with speech, language and communication impairments and emphasises our responsibility to actively develop our understanding of intervention dosage. The erosion of our clinical confidence as autonomous healthcare professionals is explored. This chapter also outlines some tentative recommendations as to a possible way of alleviating some of the tensions and conflicts between what we need to provide and what we can provide in terms of intervening in our clients' lives.

Traditionally, speech and language therapy was viewed as a health need and services were delivered accordingly either in a hospital setting or community health clinic. The primary model of intervention for children was direct (delivered by a speech and language therapist), individual, time- and context-bound. As the profession evolved and began to respond to changes, particularly in education with regard to inclusion during the nineties (DfEE, 1994, 1997, 1998; DfES, 2011), we began to explore more consultative ways of working within the school setting in response to the changing needs of the mainstream school population. Consultative or indirect models of intervention were adopted, primarily for school-aged children, which allowed larger numbers of children to receive intervention within the limited resources available. Lindsay et al. (2010) discuss the evolution of our services in relation to changes within educational policy and the emergence of more indirect models of intervention. Service models in speech and language therapy are set out in terms of several parameters by Law et al. (2002) in their critique of consultation as a model incorporating: direct versus indirect intervention; intensive versus regular input; individual versus group work; and the context, i.e., within the child's learning environment or at a clinic.

In terms of core services, that is, our first line services, our intervention options tend to be reduced to three approaches which follow predetermined routes. These models can be categorised as distinct packages of intervention. The first is *direct* speech and language therapy, which in the UK is usually a weekly, 30-minute session of therapy delivered either on an individual basis or in a group by a speech and language therapist and time-defined. The customary maximum number of therapy sessions is six, totalling three hours of intervention. The second is the *review* or "*wait and see*" approach, which allows the speech and language therapist to monitor progress without intervention over time. In this model, clients are typically offered a one-off appointment every three to six months and ideas of activities to carry out between reviews may be given to parents/carers but not actively supported by the speech and language therapist. Thirdly, there is *indirect intervention*, usually intervention delivered via a third party, where the speech and language therapist writes a programme of activities and a key person in the person's life carries out the activities as often as is required with or without the modelling of activities. This model may also include the training of others. The term "*consultative*" is often used interchangeably to describe this model.

For the large majority of our paediatric clients and families, their first experience of engaging with our services involves the application of one or other of these models of intervention. Regardless of the service to which the child or young person is attached, be it a community health clinic, a nursery or a mainstream school, the level of severity of need, or the clinical profile of the child, these models are widely applied as a way to systemise large caseloads and ensure that all clients referred to the services are on paper, at least, receiving a package of intervention or review. This is the received wisdom that prevails within paediatric speech and language therapy in the UK.

Evidence-based practice

Even a cursory review of the literature with regard to studies into the effectiveness of different paediatric speech and language interventions immediately presents a conflict with regard to evidence-based practice and the current service delivery options outlined above. In terms of research into the effectiveness of speech and language therapy intervention which targets expressive grammar, for example, we immediately see a discrepancy in dosage between what core services currently offer as direct intervention and those tested in these studies. Intervention studies into the effectiveness of shape-coding as a therapeutic technique, for example, have involved dosage levels which are consistently higher than the standard direct model of intervention. Significant treatment effects reported for comprehension of coordinating conjunctions involved four hours of direct intervention, therapy targeting comprehension of passives and Wh- questions involved 10 hours of therapy on passives and 20 hours of intervention on Wh- questions whilst comprehension of dative and Wh- comparative questions involved 10 hours of intervention (Ebbels and van der Lely 2001; Ebbels 2007, 2013). Studies into sentence construction using a usage-based approach demonstrate significant improvement with dose frequency and duration exceeding the limits of the prescribed model of direct intervention (Israel, Johnson and Brooks, 2000; Tomasello, 2003; Abbot-Smith and Behrens, 2006). Studies into sentence-combining intervention approaches show significant improvement with dose frequency and duration ranging from 18 sessions of 35 minutes each, 23 sessions of 10 minutes each and 30 sessions of 25 minutes each, way over and above the maximum dosage on offer in most core services (Saddler and Graham, 2005; Saddler et al., 2008a, b). Phillips (2014) also demonstrates significant positive results in expressive grammar and oral comprehension following an intervention programme delivered weekly over the course of 12 weeks.

If we consider studies into therapy techniques which target reading comprehension and inferencing skills such as visualising and verbalising (Bell, 1991), oral language approaches (Cain and Oakhill, 2007; Bowyer-Crane et al., 2008; Hulme and Snowling, 2011; Paul and Norbury, 2012; Snowling and Hulme, 2012) and inference training (Cain, 2010) we see a similar trend; the obvious gap in terms of level of intensity of dosage between what has been tested and what we currently offer as part of our core services has not been tested. Johnson-Glenberg (2000, 2007) investigated the effectiveness of a visualising and verbalising programme in targeting reading comprehension skills for ten 30 minute sessions over the course of 10 weeks totalling 13 hours which showed significant results. Carroll et al. (2011) investigated the effectiveness of oral language techniques in reading comprehension difficulties which involved therapy delivered for 30 minute sessions twice weekly in groups and 20 minutes a week twice a week 1:1 for a 20-week period and showed significant gains for primary-aged children. Similar issues in dosage in comparison to prescribed levels of intensity can be traced in other intervention studies. Children who received a narrative intervention programme (Joffe, 2006) showed significant gains having attended 18 lessons, three sessions weekly over six weeks in the areas of storytelling and vocabulary development. Given that 78% of speech and language therapists in the UK use a narrative-based intervention for primary-aged children with language impairments (DfE, 2012) and given that the evidence base in this intervention involves more hours, more frequently (Boudreau and Hedberg, 1999; McGregor, 2000; Hayward and Schneider, 2000; Shanks and Rippon, 2003; Shanks, 2013) then we need to seriously consider how we provide intervention targeting this clinical area. In terms of pragmatics therapy, the Social Communication Intervention Project (SCIP) is well evidenced and has shown significant treatment effects for children between the ages of 6 and 11 in the areas of social communication and conversational skills (Adams, 2008; Adams et al., 2012; Baxendale et al., 2012; Adams, 2013). This intervention programme involves 20 sessions, each an hour long, up to three times per week. One interesting point to note is a large-scale study in mental health services conducted by Timko et al. (2005, cited in Enderby, 2012) which identified the need for more intensive intervention where there was a dual diagnosis and increased severity of need. This thinking has also been explored by John (2001, cited in Enderby, 2012) within the field of speech and language therapy in terms of complexity of clinical profile; where two domains were impaired, there was a requirement for more intensive dosage of therapy. As a profession, our evidence base into the effectiveness of different intervention techniques and programmes targeting different areas of speech and language impairments is increasing rapidly. In the context of this growing evidence, we have a professional responsibility to review the use of prescribed and untested variables in relation to intervention dosage.

It needs to be acknowledged that the issue of dosage is not a simple one and there are many potential factors at play in determining the treatment effects of different components of intervention. Zeng, Law and Lindsay (2012) analysed the links between treatment effect size, dosage and intensity of intervention in 20 randomised controlled trials (RCTs). They highlight the imbalance of how little attention is paid to the issue within the field of speech and language therapy and stress the importance that, in order to develop our understanding further, both speech and language therapists and researchers should be "testing out whether extending intervention periods or intensity leads to better outcomes" (Zeng et al., 2012, pp.475-476). They recommend the need to be able to explore dosage variables such as dose form, frequency, duration and intensity where it refers to total number of teaching episodes, in relation to treatment outcomes. Yoder, Fey and Warren (2012) also highlight in their commentary the importance of unpicking the factors which potentially impact on treatment outcomes in terms of intensity, following a study they carried out into the effectiveness of early communication intervention for children with developmental delay. They conclude that we have made little or no progress in our understanding of dosage and treatment effects.

This lack of development in our knowledge base may at least partly be explained by the fact that the overwhelming majority of practising speech and language therapists work within the NHS across the UK, most of whom do not have the clinical autonomy to prescribe treatment frequency, duration or intensity. There is little consensus amongst speech and language therapists about how much intervention is optimal for children with speech language and communication needs, partly because we are not able to test our hypotheses out and gather data systematically on this issue as a result of the application of prescribed intervention models. We suspect that it is not necessarily the case that more is better (Warren and Fey, 2014). According to Yoder et al. (2012), the spacing of teaching episodes may in fact be a more critical factor in achieving best outcomes than dose frequency; however, without the clinical freedom to test these issues, our understanding will not develop.

It is inexplicable that limited resourcing is often used as a justification for capping the treatment dosage in the delivery of speech and language therapy services. That there is a finite level of resource available in the provision of services within the NHS is accepted. That these resources need to be carefully managed is obvious. As a result of the growing evidence base of significant treatment effects for specific speech and language therapy interventions or programmes such as those outlined above, however, it must be argued that to provide an untested dosage for a specific clinical profile, where we know evidence exists for a tested dosage for this profile of need, represents an unjustifiable *waste* of the limited resources available. This is not simply an argument for more speech and language therapy funding, but more to highlight that the current practice of untested dosage is no longer justifiable in terms of value for money. In medicine or pharmacy, for example, an intervention would not be recommended at an untested or reduced dosage. The National

Institute for Health and Care Excellence was set up in the UK to ensure that, within health sciences, intervention benefits were analysed in relation to their cost in order to ensure the most effective use of resources. Very few studies into the cost effectiveness of different interventions in speech and language therapy exist (Beecham et al., 2012). Boyle et al. (2007) carried out a cost benefit analysis of direct versus indirect speech and language therapy intervention delivered either in a group or individually. They concluded that group therapy delivered by a speech and language therapist showed maximum gain as measured on standardised language scores in relation to cost. Beecham et al. (2012) present a four-stage model for unit cost estimation and provide a 'checklist' of data items that should be collected about any intervention being evaluated. The use of models such as these are vital in developing our argument for funding for our services going forward. At present, given the current economic climate, it is surprising that any resources are allocated to paediatric speech and language therapy services at all, given our limited ability to present an argument of benefit of outcomes in relation to cost.

The first step for us in order to be able to develop our thinking in this direction is to argue the speech and language therapist's right to prescribe intervention dosages autonomously. Where external evidence already exists which we know will achieve significant improvements for our clients, the clinical argument is strong. We can argue the need for speech and language therapy intervention, for example, for children with persistent speech, language and communication needs because we know that more intensive intervention earlier may reduce the long-term impact of the speech and language impairment on the child's self-esteem and mental health (Clegg et al., 2005, 2012; Snowling et al., 2006), literacy skills (Stothard et al., 1998; Catts et al., 2002; Glogowska et al., 2006; Harrison et al., 2009), social isolation and employability (Ruben, 2000). Where strong external evidence exists for the timeliness of a particular intervention approach and dosage for a specific domain of language or speech impairment, then this could also give us an economic argument in terms of reducing costs to services later. For the cases where strong external evidence is not yet available, then we need to be proactive in developing hypotheses and testing these out, being careful to record specific detailed information about such factors as spacing of teaching episodes and other dosage variables so that we can develop our thinking on this. We can only do this by being able to prescribe intervention models autonomously.

We have much work to do in establishing optimal dosages for particular clinical profiles. Not only are these prescribed levels of intensity in specific incidences contrary to the evidence available to us and this therefore has direct implications for the outcomes of our clients, the use of them also presents an impediment to the development of our understanding, knowledge and thinking around dosage issues.

If little evidence exists in support of prescribed levels of dosage of direct intervention of less than three hours over the course of a block of treatment regardless of clinical profile or level of impairment, then even less exists to support a purely 'consultative' model. Whilst consultation and collaboration are equally cited in our scope of practice as values which should underpin our work, these, I believe, should remain just that; the direct translation of those values into a stand-alone model of intervention in its own right does not hold up to scrutiny. Speech and language therapy services followed the agenda of educational psychology services in developing this model of intervention which is explored fully in Law et al. (2002), who highlight concerns from speech and language therapists with regard to the application of this model and the factors which need to be in place in order for such a model to be effective. Over a decade later, we are, as a profession, still delivering this model. Certainly few robust studies exist that demonstrate significant positive outcomes for specific clinical profiles for those cases who receive a consultative model only. Whilst in research, consultative models often involve extensive training of others with direct modelling of activities and close monitoring of progress through working with, for example, parents or nursery staff, the clinical reality of such a model at times in practice, amounts to nothing more than a written programme of activities sent alongside a review report following a school visit to a class teacher. Does this constitute an intervention package? Gallagher and Chiat (2009) investigated direct versus consultative models of intervention for preschool children with specific language impairment (SLI) and found no significant differences pre- and post-therapy for the consultative group in comparison to the group who received intervention delivered by a speech and language therapist.

What is interesting is the fact that, as a profession, we have become increasingly comfortable over the last 20 years with 'handing over' the professional responsibility for our clients to another with the expectation that this person, be it a teacher, a speech and language therapy assistant (SLTA) or a learning support assistant (LSA) will have the time, ability or inclination to deliver such a programme in the absence of convincing evidence of effective outcomes. Ten years ago, Lindsay and Dockrell (2004) asked "Whose job is it?" and we still don't seem to have taken on board the parental concerns highlighted in this article. We continue to deliver this as an 'intervention' model. The assumption that it is an appropriate model in meeting the speech and language needs of, for example, children with special education needs in mainstream schools is certainly questioned by parents and researchers alike (Law et al., 2002; Lindsay and Dockrell, 2004), whereas Noell and Witt (1996) provide a comprehensive critique of the main assumptions underlying consultative models of intervention in schools. Unlike, say, a flowchart for a medical procedure, carrying out effective therapy tasks, no matter how 'procedural', involves an element in which the practitioner needs to be able to monitor and respond to the individual's response to tasks, making them harder or easier in certain specific dimensions, based on their knowledge and interpretation of the nature of the child's speech and language impairment in order to achieve a specific task response. The expectation of the knowledge of a theoretical context or framework within which to review the response to intervention is clearly an inappropriately held one in the case of an SLTA or LSA given that we know that this on-line thinking skill takes the speech and language therapist student several very intense repeated clinical learning opportunities to master. The setting of a task based on the combination of a theoretical and a client-centred rationale and then the subsequent analysis of the task response and then in turn the speech and language therapist's response to this is exactly what facilitates the process of change within the child's speech and language system. Why, therefore, do we assume that a written programme of a list of activities to be carried out without the analysis of the response of the child to the task will yield effective outcomes without the mechanism for the facilitation of change?

The point is not that training of those in a child's communication environment is not important – clearly it is vital to our outcomes – but where it takes the place of direct work with a speech and language therapist as a stand-alone 'intervention' is questionable as a practice within the context of evidence-based service delivery. A similar argument can be made for the review and monitoring of cases. This is an important aspect to our work and involves gathering baselines and reviewing progress over time. Clearly, if we did not actively review progress, we would not be able to make clinical decisions about the necessity for intervention. We certainly need a *process* of review in order to do so. The direct translation of a key process as part of our therapeutic work as an 'either/or' intervention model option is one which also needs to be scrutinised.

Responsive services

Despite our very best intentions, we still deliver a 'therapist-centred' model of service delivery as evidenced by the continued application of prescribed models of intervention which render us unable to respond to the child's individual clinical profile and needs nor the family's ability to engage. In terms of the individual profile of need, the identification of speech, language and communication disorders is agreed to be a dynamic and complex process. Lindsay et al. (2008), amongst others, highlight the process as being a function of external demands which changes over time, thereby making it difficult to develop a simple diagnostic model (Bishop, 2004; Lindsay et al., 2008; Reilly et al., 2014). How can predetermined, inflexible models of intervention be responsive to the individual needs of children with such different and changing profiles? For as long as we apply them, not only do they have a direct implication on client outcomes, they also define and limit our ability to work in equal partnership with families. Whilst we do *believe* in partnership with our families, for as long as we predetermine their needs, we are still holding control of service-planning and the decision-making power in our relationships with them. The reason we do so is not, I believe, a power issue inherent within us as speech and language therapists but more possibly to do with our passivity in terms of response to the system in which we work which has, in effect, overstepped the mark in dictating how our practice should be. The continued delivery of prescribed models of intervention is just one symptom of this expert model which assumes a predetermined need before the client and family even turn up in the clinic waiting room.

From the parent/carer perspective, attending a speech and language therapy initial appointment in which one discloses an entire personal history, one's fears and anxieties, self-doubt and guilt, hopes and expectation as a parent and in which you are leaving the appointment potentially with everything having changed *is* an individual process, one which involves loss and grief. How can we expect, in three months' time, having sent that family off unsupported following the initial contact, that they will want to or be ready to attend and engage for another one-off appointment? How can we decide unilaterally when that family is ready to engage in the therapeutic process? How can that parent and child feel anything other than that something has been 'done' to them? These issues at an individual child and family level and the language used within health systems which indicate we are still effectively a paternalistic service is explored very thoroughly in Chapter 9 of this book and so will not be explored further here. Our values and beliefs as a profession are also explored in Chapter 7 with regard to cultural responsiveness. Suffice it to say that out of the 2200 speech-language pathologists who participated in a study carried out by Watts Pappas et al. (2008), 98% reported that they agreed or strongly agreed with parental involvement in intervention, yet only 17% of the respondents gave parents the option of being involved in the service delivery format provided for their child. This gap between our beliefs and our practice is evidence of an external interference which is impacting on our ability to engage with our clients in the manner in which we believe we should: as equal partners. It represents an enormous conflict, but only one of many that we navigate daily as speech and language therapists within a large public health system attempting to respond to ever-changing political agendas in the context of ever-limited resourcing. Polmanteer and Turbiville (2000) ask who exactly the system serves and propose an answer: the system itself. Certainly not, it would seem, the family or child.

McAllister et al. (2013) explored parental and speech and language therapist expectations and experiences of paediatric speech and language therapy services in New South Wales, Australia, and highlight some interesting perceptions. They identify that parents experience significant difficulty in accessing services for their child and, by the time they do receive intervention, they are (presumably) so disempowered that they happily hand over control to the speech and language therapist. They also highlight that parents want their child to be seen by a qualified expert and prefer 1:1 intervention over groups or 'outreach' services. A similar finding is reported in Baxendale and Hesketh (2003) when comparing the effectiveness of traditional speech and language therapy intervention model and a Hanen group intervention with a strong parental preference for individual intervention as opposed to the group input. Lindsay and Dockrell (2004) highlight parental concern with the consultative model of intervention in meeting their children's speech and language therapy needs in mainstream school. Are we listening and responding? We can't, I would argue, as long as prescribed models of intervention are policy.

Whilst we can track the emergence of these prescribed models of intervention as a top-down strategy for dealing with an overstretched service, it is difficult to understand why we continue to adhere to them, in light of a growing evidence base and the increasing ease with which we can access and apply that evidence in our clinical decision making. Given the work of the Communication Trust (www.thecommunicationtrust.org.uk) and the Better Communication Research Programme (Lindsay et al., 2012), for example, there is more and more of an imperative for us to review unevidenced practice. Despite these changes in the accessibility of readily appraised evidence, we continue to absolve ourselves of our responsibilities in terms of reviewing their continued use. Why don't we listen to our 'inner' conflicts about expert-led services and practices such as these and actively reject them? Clearly, they bring a benefit to us which outweigh the risks of poor outcomes for our clients. I suggest they provide us with a structure to make sense of a perceived overwhelming 'demand' which may or may not be real from parents for intervention intensities which we believe we cannot deliver. This is not to say that at the level of the individual speech and language therapist, being the sole speech and language therapist responsible for the speech and language needs of hundreds of names on a waiting list, two days per week in a local health centre is not very real and panic inducing; it is more a comment aimed at the system where a lot of energy and resource is spent setting up administrative processes in order to try to control access to services which might be better spent on the reverse; engaging with clients.

In McAllister et al. (2011), other barriers to accessing speech and language therapy for parents, aside from the predicted ones of waiting times, distance to appointments and times of appointments, included factors such as 'readiness' for therapy. These factors resulted in only a third of referred parents being able to engage in the therapeutic process over the course of the study. If speech and language therapists were given the scope by the system in which they work to listen to their families' needs at any given time, they might discover that demand for their limited time has its own momentum which results in those families engaging in different ways, at different times in a continuum or series of interventions (Roulstone and Enderby, 2010) rather than us attempting to control access to services by intervening in an 'episodic' way when the system dictates. Roulstone et al. (2010 p. 294) state that parents look for "honesty and openness in their dealings with professionals" and are "not always seeking ever more therapy", referring to James (2008 cited in Roulstone, 2010, p.294) who also highlights this point. Enderby (2012) raises the issue that researchers were surprised to find, in a large-scale randomised control trial (RCT) of speech and language therapy service outcomes carried out in 2000 in which cases were randomly allocated to a *'therapy now'* group and a *'therapy later'* group, that parents did not want to participate in the study. This was not for the reason we might predict, i.e., that they might be allocated to the 'therapy later' group, but in fact that they could be allocated to the *'therapy now'* group (Glogowska et al., 2000). What if we were to face our greatest fear and open up our services without the need for the protection and control of a myriad administrative processes? We might not find parents and clients 'howling in the corridors' after all (Hersh, 2010, cited in Roulstone and Enderby, 2010, p.294).

Professional conflicts and ethical dilemmas

I believe that the majority of the profession works within a system which inappropriately interferes with our ability to prescribe treatment based on clinical reasoning and which is, at times, in direct conflict with our core values as a profession and therefore is harmful to our sense of clinical autonomy. Psychologically, several things happen to us, not simply explained by the professional exhaustion we feel day to day, in order to cope with these conflicts. I suggest there is a cumulative negative impact on our ability to think critically. At the beginning, as a newly-qualified speech and language therapist, you question everything. This takes time. Your manager is worried about throughput because they are answerable to some statistical measures decided upon further up the chain, and when they are not worrying about throughput, they spend considerable energy dealing with irate users of the service. Your first appraisal focus is about how to prioritise cases based on protocol and to develop your time management skills. The net result of resource-led prioritisation protocols and workload pressures is that you don't have the time to undergo the important questioning processes you need to in order to maintain your critical thinking skills. These skills, needless to say, were well developed to begin with. Because you are newly-qualified and lacking confidence in your own clinical judgement, you adhere to these prioritisation protocols even though you know these are not evidenced. You know this because you have spent anything between two years post degree and four years as an undergraduate, reading this literature. After a while, just doing and not critically appraising results in a blurring of the boundaries between your clinical opinion and the services that the system offers. We in effect begin to own the system. We begin to find protection within the system. We begin to accept and perpetuate the implicit unspoken values and judgements of the system, the received wisdoms of the professional culture. Every day we hear terms such as 'difficult families' (those who argue for more intervention for their child), 'poor/non-attenders' (those who for whatever reason are not able to commit to coming to appointments at a particular time with extremely valid reasons but who don't get a chance to express these reasons and are therefore discharged from services), and after a while we stop flinching. The system allows us to deflect and keep at arm's length the enormous ethical dilemmas which arise when we do intervene in clients' lives in what we know and believe to be an 'insufficient' way. Then when the few families that can engage on our terms do, we hear ourselves using justifications or unfounded rationales for the limited services we can deliver.

An example of this would be the idea of a 'period of consolidation'. This concept is very often quoted by speech and language therapists to clients as a rationale for a 'break' from the therapeutic process. The introduction of the concept to parents/carers and clients usually coincides with the end of a prescribed block of treatment when a decision is made (by the speech and language therapist) about whether the child needs further intervention. Whilst consolidation in relation to learning theory in neuropsychology refers to a process during the period of time subsequent to an educational event which is understood to influence our ability to develop our memory skills, there is no evidence in the literature that a process of consolidation occurs in the period after we finish a speech and language therapy intervention block that is beneficial in terms of the maintenance of skills learned. It is a concept which we continue to share with our clients and families as though it will somehow strengthen the positive outcomes of therapy. It is also a way of avoiding other more difficult conversations.

Deciding when intervention should cease is one of the most complicated, ethically loaded and emotionally laden procesess in the therapeutic relationship as explored by Hersh (2010), Roulstone and Enderby (2010) and Quattlebaum and Steppling (2010). In paediatric speech and language therapy services, the system allows us to bypass that thinking by prescribing the beginning and end of our engagement in client's lives in six-weekly blocks. Speech and language therapists in the private and non-maintained sectors rarely use terms such as 'consolidation' as a rationale for ceasing the provision of services. Rather, they are in a position to make an autonomous clinical decision and therefore to consider a whole host of complex factors such as clinical profile, client motivation for therapy, response to therapy and rate of progress versus expected rate of progress, external life factors amongst others which may affect the family and child's ability to engage with the therapeutic process. I disagree with the idea that it is helpful to speech and language therapists to provide structure in the form of prescribed packages of care that lessen their feelings of personal responsibility (Roulstone and Enderby, 2010) because I believe when we stop feeling responsible, we should no longer have the right to intervene in people's lives.

Some recommendations

As a starting point, I suggest we urgently need to critically appraise our practice in relation to how we intervene in families' lives in order to achieve the best outcomes for the child with speech, language and communication needs. We need to abandon prescribed models of intervention and trial dosage variables. We need to access support and advice from researchers about ways of systematically collecting data in relation to the delivery of intervention to ensure we are taking into account the characteristics of dosage which might have the most important impact on outcomes. We also need to be more honest with our clients about the limits of what we can offer. In the longer term, as a profession, we have ongoing work to do in rediscovering our clinical autonomy.

Gabbay and Le May (2004) studied decision-making practices of GPs and practice nurses and concluded that the most powerful influence on clinical decision making was local policy mediated by organisational demands and constraints. I would argue that as a profession, we need to take a step back and analyse our clinical decision-making influences. We need to redress the imbalance of the weighting that local policy has on our practice if it demands that we deliver untested treatment dosages or impedes our ability to work in partnership with our clients. We need to reject, on our clients' behalf, the implicit values which lead to defensive practice. We need to take back the power of clinical decision making in our professional lives from those who drive the health service agenda. We need to be clear about the factors which are influencing our decision making. Our work as speech and language therapists is powerful, rewarding and vital. It is a privilege to be able to intervene in people's lives. Our clinical decision making as a process is agreed to involve a multitude of influencing factors and requires complex thinking. I believe we have lost touch with our clinical autonomy. We urgently need to rediscover this as a first step.

We then need to respect our clients sufficiently to be clear about which decisions are, in the main, resource-led and those which are made from a clinical perspective. If you went to your GP and he/she prescribed only half a course of antibiotics due to limited resources but didn't explain that it was only a half a course of antibiotics after which you won't feel any better, would you be happy with this service? If the GP explained that he/she didn't know whether these would effect any health improvements as they had not been tested at this dosage, but you should try them anyway because he/she had seen some improvements for other clients with similar symptoms previously, what does this do to the dynamic? It's not so much whether you would in the end decide to take the antibiotics or not, but how honesty on the part of the clinician would have two effects; it gives the power back to the client in making the decision about intervention and it empowers the clinician by maintaining critical distance between themselves and the system. Is this something we do for our clients and families when they become involved in our services? If we are truly working in partnership, why is so much left unsaid when families first engage with us? We should be having honest conversations with our clients around the intervention packages that we offer and others that we don't or can't but are also available whilst having even more difficult conversations with policy makers higher up the chain about being able to deliver the most effective model of intervention. Where we are delivering intervention that is not evidence-based but resource-led, then as practising clinicians we need to be clear in our own minds about the difference, and this needs to be part of an explicit conversation with our clients at the point where we are about to engage them in a block of intervention.

Enderby (2012) asked the very pertinent question *"How much therapy is enough?"* and discussed the very complex issues in determining an answer. How far further are we in answering this vital question in terms of effectiveness of intervention for our clients, for our families fighting for services, for GPs, health visitors and the teachers who refer to us, in communicating to the lawyers that fight for families to secure speech and language therapy services, for tribunal judges who make a decision about services, for the health economists who need to ensure cost effectiveness and for the politicians to understand the importance of what we do? The issues highlighted in this chapter are not only the obvious conflicts which arise for us in terms of client outcomes when we deliver predetermined models of intervention, but for as long as we do, we stop having honest conversations with the families we serve and we limit ourselves in being able to develop our understanding of the complexities of dosage across different client groups. The implication of that final impact is far reaching, in that it impedes our ability to develop a strong argument in favour of funding for speech and language therapy services going forward. Let's start to take the time to ask ourselves, as a profession, some serious questions.

References

Abbot-Smith, K. & Behrens, H. (2006) How known constructions influence the acquisition of other constructions: The German passive future constructions. *Cognitive Science*, 30, 995–1026.

Adams, C. (2008) Intervention for children with pragmatic language impairments. In C. Norbury, J. Tomlin and D. Bishop (Eds) *Understanding Developmental Language Disorders: From Theory to Practice*. Sussex: Psychology Press, pp.189–204.

Adams, C. (2013) Social Communication Intervention Project: An evidence-based programme for school aged children. Available at: www.psychsci.manchester.ac.uk/ scip/conferencepresentations/ASLTIPmarch2013pdf

Adams, C., Lockton, E., Freed, J., Gaile, J., Earl, G., McBean, K. & Law, J. (2012) The Social Communication Intervention Project: A randomized controlled trial of the effectiveness of speech and language therapy for school-age children who have pragmatic and social communication problems with or without autism spectrum disorder. *International Journal of Language & Communication Disorders*, 47(3), 233–244.

Allen, J. & Marshall, C.R. (2011) Parent-Child Interaction Therapy (PCIT) in school-aged children with specific language impairment. *International Journal of Language & Communication Disorders*, 46(4), 397–410.

American Speech-Language-Hearing Association (2008a) Core knowledge and skills in early intervention speech-language pathology practice. www.asha.org/policy.

American Speech-Language-Hearing Association (2008b) Roles and responsibilities of Speech-Language Pathologists in early intervention: Guidelines. www.asha.org/policy.

American Speech-Language-Hearing Association (2008c) Roles and responsibilities of Speech-Language Pathologist in early intervention: Position Paper. www.asha.org/policy.

American Speech-Language-Hearing Association (2008d) Roles and responsibilities of Speech-Language Pathologist in early intervention: Technical Report. www.asha.org/policy.

Baxendale, J. & Hesketh, A. (2003) Comparison of the effectiveness of the Hanen Parent Programme and traditional therapy. *International Journal of Language & Communication Disorders*, 38(4), 397–415.

Baxendale, J., Lockton, E., Adams, C. & Gaile, J. (2012) Parent and teacher perceptions of participation and outcomes in an intensive communication intervention for children with pragmatic language impairment. *International Journal of Language & Communication Disorders*, 48(1), 41–53.

Beecham, J., Law, J., Zeng, B. & Lindsay, G. (2012) Costing children's speech, language and communication interventions. *International Journal of Language & Communication Disorders*, 47(5), 477–486.

Bell, N. (1991) *Visualizing and Verbalizing: For Language Comprehension and Thinking*. Darien, CT: Lindamoodbell.

Bishop, D.V.M. (2004) Specific language impairment: diagnostic dilemma. In Hans Van Balkom and L. Verhoeven, *Classification of Developmental Language Disorders: Theoretical Issues and Clinical Implications*. Hillsdale, N.J: Lawrence Erlbaum, pp.309–326.

Boudreau, D.M. & Hedberg, N.L. (1999) A comparison of early literacy skills in children with specific language impairment and their typically developing peers. *American Journal of Speech-Language Pathology*, 8, 249–260.

Bowyer-Crane, C., Snowling, M., Duff, F., Fieldsend, E., Carroll, J., Miles, J. & Hulme, C. (2008) Improving early language and literacy skills: Differential effects of an oral language versus a phonology with reading intervention. *Journal of Child Psychology and Psychiatry and Allied Disciplines*, 49(4), 422–432.

Boyle, J., McCartney, E., Forbes, J. and O'Hare, A. (2007) A randomised controlled trial and economic evaluation of direct versus indirect and individual versus group modes of speech and language therapy for children with primary language impairment. *Health Technology Assessment*; 11(25), 1–139.

Cain, K. (2010) *Reading Development and Difficulties*. Oxford: Wiley-Blackwell.

Cain, K. & Oakhill, J. (Eds) (2007) *Children's Comprehension Problems in Oral and Written Language*. New York: Guilford Press.

Carroll, J.M., Bowyer-Crane, C., Duff, F., Hulme, C. & Snowling, M.J. (2011) *Effective Intervention for Language and Literacy in the Early Years*. Oxford: Wiley-Blackwell.

Catts, H.W., Fey, M.E., Tomlin, J.B. & Zhang, X. (2002) A longitudinal study of reading outcomes in children with language impairments. *Journal of Speech, Language and Hearing Research*, 45, 1145–1157.

Clegg, J., Hollis,,C., Mawhood, L. & Rutter, M. (2005) Developmental language disorders: A follow-up in later adult life: Cognitive, language and psychosocial outcomes. *Journal of Child Psychology and Psychiatry*, 46, 128–149.

Clegg, J., Ansorge, L., Stackhouse, J. & Donlan, C. (2012) Developmental communication impairments in adults: Outcomes and life experiences of the adults and their parents. *Language, Speech Hearing Services in Schools*, 43, 521–535.

Department for Education and Employment (1994) *The Code of Practice on the Identification and Assessment of Special Educational Needs*. Nottingham: DfES.

Department for Education and Skills (1997) *Excellence for All Children: Meeting Special Educational Needs: A Programme of Action*. London: HMSO.

Department for Education and Skills (1998) *Meeting Special Educational Needs: A Programme of Action*. London: HMSO.

Department for Education and Skills (2001) *Special Educational Needs Code of Practice*. Nottingham: DfES.

Department for Education (2012) *Exploring Interventions for Children and Young People with Speech, Language and Communication Needs: A Study of Practice.* Available at www.gov.uk

Dockrell, J., Lindsay, G., Letchford, B. & Mackie, C. (2006) Educational provision for children with specific speech and language difficulties: Perspectives of speech and language therapy service managers. *International Journal of Language & Communication Disorders,* 41(4), 423–440.

Ebbels, S. (2007). Teaching grammar to school-aged children with specific language impairment using Shape Coding. *Child Language Teaching & Therapy,* 23(1), 67–93.

Ebbels, S. (2013) Effectiveness of intervention for grammar in school-aged children with primary language impairments: A review of the evidence. *Child Language, Teaching and Therapy,* 30(1), 7–40.

Ebbels, S. & van der Lely, H. (2001) Meta-syntactic therapy using visual coding for children with severe persistent SLI. *International Journal of Language & Communication Disorders,* 36 (supplement), 345–350.

Enderby, P. (2012) How much therapy is enough? The impossible question! *International Journal of Speech-Language Pathology,* 14(5), 432–437.

Fey, M. (2006) Clinical forum. Commentary on "Making evidence-based decisions about child language intervention in schools" by Gillam S.L. and Gillam R.B. *Language, Speech & Hearing Services in Schools,* 37(4), 316–319.

Fey, M., Yoder, P., Warren, S., Bredin-Oja, S., Oetting, J. & Crais, E. (2013) Is more better? Milieu communication teaching in toddlers with intellectual disabilities. *Journal of Speech, Language & Hearing Research,* 56(2), 679–693.

Gabbay, J. & Le May, A. (2004) Evidence based guidelines or collectively constructed "mindlines"? Ethnographic study of knowledge management in primary care. *British Medical Journal,* 329, 1013–1016.

Gallagher, A. & Chiat, S. (2009) Evaluation of speech and language therapy interventions for pre-school children with specific language impairment: A comparison of outcomes following specialist intensive, nursery-based and no intervention. *International Journal of Language & Communication Disorders,* 44(5), 616–638.

Glogowska, M., Roulstone, S., Enderby, P. & Peters, T.J. (2000) Randomised controlled trial of community based speech and language therapy in preschool children. *British Medical Journal,* 321(7266), 923–926.

Glogowska, M., Roulstone, S., Peters, T. & Enderby, P. (2006) Early speech- and language-impaired children: Linguistic, literacy, and social outcomes. *Developmental Medicine and Child Neurology,* 48(6), 489–494.

Harrison, L.J., Mc Leod, S., Berthelson, D. & Walker, S. (2009) Literacy, numeracy and learning in school-aged children identified as having speech and language impairment in early childhood. *International Journal of Speech-Language Pathology,* 11, 392–403.

Hayward, D. & Schneider, P. (2000) Effectiveness of teaching story grammar knowledge to pre-school children with language impairment. An exploratory study. *Child Language, Teaching and Therapy,* 16(3), 255–284.

Hersh, D. (2010) I can't sleep at night with discharging this lady: The personal impact of ending therapy on speech-language pathologists. *International Journal of Speech-Language Pathology,* 12(4), 283–291.

Hulme, C. & Snowling, M. (2011) Children's reading comprehension difficulties: Nature, causes, and treatments. *Psychological Sciences,* 20(3), 139–142.

Israel, M., Johnson, C. & Brooks, P. J. (2000) From states to events: The acquisition of English passive participles. *Cognitive Linguistics,* 11(1/2), 103–129.

Joffe, V. (2006) Enhancing language and communication in language-impaired secondary school-aged children. In J. Clegg & J. Ginsborg (Eds), *Language and Social Disadvantage: Theory Into Practice.* Chichester: John Wiley & Sons, pp.207–216.

Johnson-Glenberg, M. (2000) Training reading comprehension in adequate decoders/ poor comprehenders: Verbal versus visual strategies. *Journal of Educational Psychology,* 92(4), 772–782.

Johnson-Glenberg, M. (2007) Web-based reading comprehension instruction: Three studies of 3-D readers. In McNamara, D. (Ed.), *Reading Comprehension Strategies: Theories, Interventions and Technolo*gies. New York: Lawrence Erlbaum Associates, pp.293–324.

Law, J., Lindsay, G., Peacey, N., Gascoigne, M., Soloff, N., Radford, J. & Band, S. (2002) Consultation as a model for providing speech and language therapy in schools: A panacea or one step too far? Papers from the 7th European Congress of Psychology. *Child Language Teaching & Therapy,* 18(2), 145–163.

Lindsay, G. & Dockrell, J. (2004) Whose job is it? Parents' concerns about the needs of their children with language problems. *Journal of Special Education,* 37(4), 225–235.

Lindsay, G., Desforges, M., Dockrell, J., Law, J., Peacey, N. & Beecham, J. (2008) *Effective and Efficient Use of Resources in Services for Children and Young People with Speech, Language and Communication Needs.* RW053. Nottingham: DCSF.

Lindsay, G., Dockrell, J., Desforges, M., Law, J. & Peacey, N. (2010) Meeting the needs of children and young people with speech, language and communication difficulties. *International Journal of Language & Communication Disorders,* 45(4), 448–460.

Lindsay, G., Dockrell, J., Law, J., & Roulstone, S. (2012). Better communication research programme: Improving provision for children and young people with speech, language and communication needs. London: DfE.

McAllister, L., McCormack, J., McLeod, S. & Harrison, L.J. (2011) Expectations and experiences of accessing and participation in services for childhood speech and impairment. *International Journal of Speech-Language Pathology,* 13(3), 251–267.

McGregor, K.K. (2000) The development and the enhancement of narrative skills in a preschool classroom towards a solution to clinician-client mismatch. *American Journal of Speech-Language Pathology*, 9, 55–71.

Noell, G.H. & Witt, J.C. (1996) A critical re-evaluation of five fundamental assumptions underlying behavioural consultation. *School Psychology Quarterly*, 11, 189–203.

Paul, R. & Norbury, C. (2012) *Language Disorders from Infancy Through Adolescence: Listening, Speaking, Reading, Writing and Communicating*, 4th ed. St Louis, Mo.: Elsevier.

Paul, D. & Roth, F.P. (2011) Guiding principles and clinical applications for speech-language pathology practice in early intervention. *Language, Speech & Hearing Services in Schools*, 42(3), 320–330.

Phillips, B. (2014) Promotion of syntactical development and oral comprehension: Development and initial evaluation of a small-group intervention. *Child Language Teaching & Therapy*, 30(1), 63–77.

Polmanteer, K. & Turbiville, V. (2000) Family-responsive individualized family service plans for speech-language pathologists. *Language, Speech, and Hearing Services in Schools*, 31(1), 4–14.

Quattlebaum, P. & Steppling, M. (2010) Preparation for ending therapeutic relationships. *International Journal of Speech-Language Pathology*, 12(4), 313–316.

Reilly, S., Tomblin, B., Law, J., Mckean, C., Mensah, F.K., Morgan, A., Goldfeld, S., Nicholson, J.M. & Wak,e M. (2014) Specific Language Impairment: A convenient label for whom? *International Journal of Language and Communication Disorders*. In press.

Robertson, S.B. & Weismer, S.E. (1999) Effects of treatment on linguistic and social skills in toddlers with delayed language development. *Journal of Speech, Language & Hearing Research*, 42(5), 1234–1248.

Roulstone, S. & Enderby, P. (2010) The end of the affair: Discharging clients from speech and language pathology. *International Journal of Speech-Language Pathology*, 12(4), 292–295.

Roulstone, S. (2008) *Prioritising Child Health: Practice and Principles*. London: Routledge.

Royal College of Speech and Language Therapists (2006) *Communicating Quality 3*. Oxon: Speechmark.

Ruben, R.J. (2000) Redefining the survival of the fittest: Communication disorders in the 21st century. *Laryngoscope*, 110, 241–245.

Saddler, B. & Graham, S. (2005) The effects of peer-assisted sentence-combining instruction on the writing performance of more and less skilled young writers. *Journal of Educational Psychology*, 97(1), 43–54.

Saddler, B., Asaro, K. & Beforhooz, B. (2008a) The effects of peer-assisted sentence-combining practice on four young writers with learning disabilities. *Learning Disabilities: A Contemporary Journal*, 1(6), 17–31.

Saddler, B., Beforhooz, B. & Asaro, K.(2008b) The effects of sentence-combining instruction on the writing of fourth-grade students with writing difficulties. *The Journal of Special Education*, 42(2), 79–90.

Shanks, B. (2013) Speaking and listening through narrative. In N. Grove (Ed.), *Using Storytelling to Support Children and Adults with Special Needs: Transforming Lives Through Telling Tales*. New York: Routledge, pp. 48–55.

Shanks, B. & Rippon, H. (2003) *Speaking and Listening Through Narrative: A Pack of Activities and Ideas*, 2nd ed. Keighley, Yorkshire: Black Sheep Press.

Snowling, M. & Hulme, C. (2012) Interventions for children's language and literacy difficulties. *International Journal of Language & Communication Disorders*, 47(1), 27–34.

Snowling, M., Bishop, D., Stothard, S., Chipchase, B. & Kaplan, C. (2006) Psychosocial outcomes at 15 years of children with a preschool history of speech-language impairment. *Journal of Child Psychology and Psychiatry, and Allied Disciplines*, 47(8), 759–765.

Speech Pathology Australia (2010) *Evidence-Based Practice in Speech Pathology: Position Paper*. www.speechpathologyaustralia.org.au

Stothard, S.E., Snowling, M.J., Bishop, D.V., Chipchase, B.B. & Kaplan, C.A. (1998) Language-impaired preschoolers: A follow-up into adolescence. *Journal of Speech, Language and Hearing Research*, 41(2), 407–418.

Tomasello, M.(2003). *Constructing a Language: A Usage-based Theory of Language Acquisition*. Cambridge, MA: Harvard University Press.

Warren S. & Fey M. (2008) A randomised trial of longitudinal effects of low intensity responsivity education/prelinguistic milieu teaching. *Journal of Speech, Language & Hearing Research*, 49(3), 526–547.

Watts Pappas, N., McLeod, S., McAllister, L. & McKinnon, D.H. (2008) Parental involvement in speech intervention: A national survey. *Clinical Linguistics & Phonetics*, 22(4–5), 335–244.

Yoder, P., Fey, M. & Warren, S. (2012) Studying the impact of intensity is important but complicated. *International Journal of Speech-Language Pathology*, 14(5), 410–413.

Zeng, B., Law, J. & Lindsay, G. (2012) Characterizing optimal intervention intensity: The relationship between dosage and effect size in interventions for children with developmental speech and language difficulties. *International Journal of Speech-Language Pathology*, 14(5), 471–477.

3 Supervision in speech and language therapy; learning from other professions

Jane Stokes

Supervision in speech and language therapy is now accepted as good practice within the profession. The Royal College of Speech and Language Therapists (RCSLT) published comprehensive guidance on supervision in 2012 (www.rcslt.org). Much of this relates to the nuts and bolts of supervision: content, contracts and recording. A distinction is made between non-managerial supervision and line management supervision but although the guidance recommends that therapists should have access to both, it is not clear whether this is the case. It is my experience that this access is not universal. Sparkes and Simpson (2013) state perceptively that the role of supervision has now extended to one that "supports and facilitates emotional resilience... fosters an individual's personal/professional resources to manage change" (p.23). This constitutes a demanding role for the supervisor, who is often involved in managing his or her own responses to change at the same time as facilitating emotional resilience in the supervisee. Are we adequately trained and supported to do this in the profession?

There is limited training for speech and language therapists specifically on supervision and such that exists tends to comprise a brief two-day course with no follow-up or support. The courses are often run by the employing authorities and often focus on the process rather than the practice of supervision. More in-depth courses on supervision are not widely available across the country. There is limited specialist training focusing on the particular issues facing speech and language therapists in practice. Simpson and Sparkes published a useful series of articles (2008) and do provide training in the UK which is highly regarded (http://www.intandem.co.uk). But it is recognised that "all too often, clinicians are placed in a supervisory role with limited or no supervisory experience... achieving clinical competence does not necessarily mean one has the ability to be an effective supervisor" (Hudson in Lubinski and Hudson, 2013, p.523). Additionally, there is a lack of consensus in how supervisors should be trained. In a systematic review of training for clinical supervisors, Milne et al. (2011) found that much supervision was being practised incompetently, and there was limited evidence to suggest that the training of supervisors resulted in a change in supervision practice. There was no agreement as to what outcome measures could be used to assess competence in supervision. Follow-up support for newly-trained supervisors is limited.

Ultimately there is an aspiration that by providing safe clinical supervision the care of the client will be enhanced. Although there is an assumption made that the main purpose of providing supervision is to improve the quality of client care, there has been no research in speech and language therapy into the impact of supervision on the quality of client care. The ASHA (American Speech-Language Hearing Association) document on clinical supervision (2008) states: "... there is little empirical evidence in the area of supervision (Spence, Wilson, Kavanagh, Strong and Worrall, 2001) especially as it relates to client outcomes". Pearce et al. (2013) in their systematic review found that current research into the content of clinical supervision for nursing and allied health practitioners is limited and of low quality. They felt that further research is needed "to determine what content in clinical supervision is associated with better quality and safety, particularly for health professions other than nursing and psychology" (p.139).

So here we have an example of a tacit assumption, that clinical supervision impacts on the quality of client care, which has a limited evidence base – a familiar scenario for speech and language therapists.

It could easily be the case that in becoming a clinical supervisor the therapist may just extend his or her therapeutic role in relation to the supervisee without being aware that being a clinical supervisor is not necessarily the same as being a therapist, although some skills may be common to both roles. The skills do overlap and without skilled support it could be difficult to separate the role of therapist from the role of supervisor of a colleague.

As a team leader in NHS speech and language therapy settings I was involved in the supervision of more recently-qualified staff. I took on this role with no formal training. I had been privileged to have been supervised myself by some skilled managers and to have had access early on in my career to structured supervision from psychiatry, psychology and family therapy colleagues. I was able to use the learning from that experience to shape my supervision style and practice but I lacked any theoretical understanding of the process of clinical supervision and it is my observation that this is the case for many middle managers who take on the role of clinical supervisor within speech and language therapy. I subsequently attended a short two-day course but this was only after I had been supervising for over six years. It was only once I had left the NHS and was asked to help design a post-registration course in clinical supervision that I had the opportunity to research more about the nature of clinical supervision. I was introduced to the theoretical perspectives commonly used in occupational therapy supervision. I had time to read the literature on clinical supervision in the helping professions. This made me then realise that speech and language therapists are for the most part inadequately trained in this vital skill, are largely unaware of different models and the theoretical underpinnings, and I realised that we could do well to learn from the work done in other helping professions in developing our own supervision practice.

Some of the research on clinical supervision in speech and language therapy has focused on the role of clinical educators but much of this is relevant to supervision of qualified therapists. For example, Joshi and McAllister (1998) observe that supervisory styles may depend more on the past experience of the supervisor rather than be based on theoretical models of supervision. They mention that the difficulty in trying to analyse supervisory style may be due to the somewhat ad hoc way in which supervisory styles have developed. The ASHA document on clinical supervision (2008) refers to Dowling (2001) and McCrae and Brasseur (2003) whose research indicates that "supervisors who engage in supervisory conferences/meetings without formal supervisory training tend to dominate talk time, problem solving and strategy development". Without skilled training and supported follow up there is a danger that supervision practice falls into these ineffective patterns.

Clinical supervision in the helping professions has received more coverage in books relating to nursing and occupational therapy and it is useful for speech and language therapists to be directed to these. There are a number of theoretical models of supervision that can inform practice in speech and language therapy. Hawkins and Shohet (2012) have developed the seven-eyed model of supervision. The model was developed in order to include the different areas that can be focused on in supervision. It identifies that in any supervision situation there are at least four elements: a supervisor, a supervisee, a client and a work context. They draw attention to the fact that there are seven points of focus in the supervisory relationship:

- A focus on the client and on what and how they present
- An exploration of the strategies and interventions used by the supervisee
- An exploration of the relationship between the client and the supervisee
- A focus on the supervisee
- A focus on the relationship between supervisor and supervisee
- A focus on the supervisor's own process
- A focus on the wider contexts of work.

Additionally, there are two interlocking relationships – the supervisor–supervisee relationship and the client–supervisee relationship. Hence the supervision setting has a number of complex dynamics at play, and it is vital to be aware of these.

Importantly, Hawkins and Shohet (2012) refer to the relationship that is not in the room, the relationship between the supervisee and the client but which needs to be brought to the foreground, a process that has been called "getting the client into the room" (Hawkins and Schwenk in Bachkirova, Jackson and Clutterbuck (2011, p.30). They also emphasise that the organisational context that the supervisee works in is as worthy of attention as the supervisee and the client. There is an acknowledgement that the supervisory context may mirror the situation between the supervisee and the client. It may be the case that the dynamics that surface in the relationship between the supervisor and the supervisee may echo something that is going on in the clinical intervention itself. The discussion of this requires expert and sensitive management. There is little structured support for the process of supervision in speech and language therapy. It is not possible to acquire these skills on the job. Supervisors should themselves be given support in the process of supervision to ensure that they can develop the advanced skills required.

The key functions of supervision have been discussed by a number of authors. Proctor (2001) refers to the normative, formative and restorative aspects of supervision. The **normative** aspect refers to the situation where the supervisor accepts and shares with the supervisee the responsibility for ensuring that the supervisee's work is professional and ethical, operating within whatever codes, laws and organisational norms apply.

The **formative** aspect refers to the situation in supervision where the supervisor has a role in providing feedback that enables the supervisee to develop the skills, theoretical knowledge and personal attributes that will mean the supervisee becomes an increasingly competent practitioner. The **restorative** aspect refers to the situation where the supervisor is there to listen, support and challenge the supervisee when personal issues, doubts and insecurities arise. Speech and language therapists fulfilling the role of clinical supervisor may feel that they emphasise one of these aspects more than others. It is useful to reflect on this, and to be helped in reflecting on this by the supervisor herself accessing skilled supervision.

Kadushin (1992) talks about similar aspects but uses different terminology; he considers that supervision can fulfil three different functions:

- **Educational** – here the focus is on the educational development of the supervisee, facilitating the fulfilment of potential. The supervisor's key role is to encourage reflection on their work guiding their professional development.

- **Support** – here the focus is on both practical and psychological support to fulfil the responsibilities of the supervisee's role. It is recognised that the stress and pressure at work can take its toll and the role of the supervisor in supportive supervision is to assist in the effective management of stress.

- **Administrative/managerial** – here the focus is on the maintenance of high professional standards, and adherence to policies and procedures in the furtherance of good practice. The supervisor has a role in contributing to the quality of the supervisee's work.

Again it can be instructive to reflect on one's own supervisory experience and to explore which of these functions tend to predominate. This requires support and guidance from an experienced supervisor and time should be allocated to allow detailed reflection and feedback in these areas.

A number of models emphasise the developmental nature of supervision. Underlying these developmental models is an assumption that supervision supports our professional and personal growth. Stoltenberg and Delworth (1987) described the different stages of development, facilitated by supervision, from novice to journeyman, and then from independent craftsman to master craftsman. During this process the supervisor has to adopt different strategies and techniques to support the supervisee's growth.

Level 1, the novice level, is seen as a self-centred stage, characterised by anxiety, dependency and high motivation. At this stage, the supervisor may need to provide structure and give more prescriptive advice. At **Level 2**, the journeyman stage, the supervisee may display fluctuations between dependence and autonomy and an uncertainty about their role. At this stage according to Stoltenberg and Delworth (1987), supervisors need to provide support, clarify ambivalence and provide modelling. **Level 3**, the independent craftsman stage, is a more process-centred stage. At this stage, the supervisee is more able to move between their own responses and the client's awareness. The supervisor has a role in providing stimulation for the supervisee to continue to develop. At **Level 4**, the master craftsman stage, the focus is on the context. The supervisee is now displaying a high level of personal autonomy, and has greater insight into their own and the client's contexts. Personal and professional knowledge is integrated and synthesised.

There are many related fields that we could draw on in deepening our knowledge of clinical supervision. We could incorporate aspects of the so-called strengths-based approach to supervision in clinical practice. Edwards (2013) encourages us to view supervision as a dialectic collaborative process rather than an opportunity to set supervisees straight and fix their mistakes. This strengths-based approach to supervision is grounded in theory such as Albert Bandura's ideas of self-efficacy and personal agency, collaborative language-based therapy (Goolishian, 1990), narrative therapy (White and Epston, 1990), solution-focused therapy (de Shazer, 1994) or a resiliency model (Walsh, 2006), plus themes from positive psychology (Seligman and Csikszentmihalyi, 2000). Speech and language therapists are not exposed to this wealth of theory during training or during their career progression towards becoming a supervisor. We can learn much from theories relating to attachment; the work of McCluskey (2005) is highly relevant here. She has explored the dynamics of attachment in adult life in relation to care-givers and care-seekers. These are all approaches which could contribute to the depth and authenticity of our supervision practice but which are not widely used or applied in supervision in speech and language therapy.

As a profession we can learn a lot from the work of Harlene Anderson. Her approach challenges the notions of knowledge as objective and fixed, and favours the construction of knowledge as social, as fluid, the knower and knowledge as interdependent, knowledge as relational and the multiplicity of 'truths' (http://www.harleneanderson.org/writings).

She talks about creating a dialogical space and facilitating a dialogical process – through adopting a philosophical stance characterised by an attitude of openness to, respect for, curiosity about and connection with the other. She talks about the importance of 'not-knowing', referring to the assumption that we do not know what is best for the other person. The process is one of shared inquiry.

Anderson sees supervision as a collaborative endeavour characterised by 3 Cs: connect, collaborate and construct. Speech and language therapists may achieve this during their development as supervisors but it is important that they are allowed time to reflect and build on their skills through explicit training and support as supervisors. This is not something that we tend to prioritise within the profession. We focus on developing the service for our clients sometimes at the expense of spending time developing ourselves as supervisors and supporters of each other. Weld (2012) builds on these ideas and focuses on the fact that sensitivity and respectful curiosity should form the basis of supervision. Ferguson (2008) discusses the term 'supervision', which carries with it an intrinsic assumption of power and responsibility in the relationship which may or may not reflect the nature of the relationship (p.115). In the health professions, it is often the case that the supervisor role is taken by someone who also has a managerial role in relation to that member of staff, which can confuse the difference between non-managerial and managerial supervision. Issues of power can get involved if the supervisor is also the manager.

In exploring this area, I began to reflect on the gaps in our reflective processes within the profession, the resistance to thinking about uncomfortable aspects of our role and the fact that we are often poorly supported to deal with the affective aspects of the relationships that we develop with clients. Issues of transference and countertransference that may well occur during therapy relationships have received almost no attention in speech and language therapy literature. In nursing training, there has been much work done on the therapeutic use of self – a concept that is absent in speech and language therapy pre-registration training. The professional use of self first entered the literature around infancy and mental health when Bertacchi and Stott (1992) quoted in Fourie (2011) defined the use of self as "understanding oneself and using oneself as a vehicle for good practice" (p.197). It has been further developed and is now seen as the quality in professionals which involves paying attention to one's own inner experiences and how these interact with the other in a therapeutic relationship. As Geller in Fourie (2011) points out: learning how to manage our emotional reactions has not traditionally been part of the training in speech-language pathology (p.206). Silverman in Fourie (2011) says that we attend to the client and not necessarily, or to the same degree, to the client–clinician relationship. Geller in Fourie (2011) talks about professional use of self: "attention to the affective and intersubjective aspects of clinical relationships has been neglected in speech language pathology" (p.197) and later, "What has been neglected in speech-language pathology is an understanding of the power of relationships and the transformational impact of practitioners on clients and families (and vice versa)" (p.200). It would require skilled supervision to support practitioners to explore these issues of the clinical relationship, and it is unlikely that speech and language therapists are adequately trained to provide this. It is also not part of our accepted practice. There are a few services where colleagues from psychological therapy professions have been involved in the supervision of speech and language therapists but this could, and in my view should, become routine. How can we be effective in our relationship with clients if we are not given the space to reflect on this with a skilled supervisor?

McDonald in Fourie (2011) provides a really useful chapter on the transference relationship in speech language therapy, but this aspect of the relationship between client and therapist, and between supervisee and supervisor, has rarely been addressed, and is scarcely touched on in pre-registration training of speech and language therapists. McDonald (2011) usefully assesses the relevance of the transference relationship in speech and language therapy. She draws attention to the fact that in working with someone in a therapeutic relationship we are communicating both at a conscious and at an unconscious level. She provides useful definitions of the terms 'transference' and 'countertransference' and how they may relate to the speech and language therapy context, acknowledging that features of these processes can be subtle and difficult to identify. She also discusses projective identification. She says that, as clinicians, "... we have the potential to elicit strong transferences and counter-transferences that if understood, could be managed to ensure a safe and positive outcome; but if ignored could lead to a myriad of relational hazards" (p.173). McDonald goes on to state that clinical supervision is essential in enabling clinicians to "reflect on and to disentangle intense emotional reactions, thus ensuring safe and professional practice" (pp.179, 180). The majority of speech and language therapists are not aware of, nor do they have space to reflect on, these issues with expert professional support. Norman-Murch (1996) cited in Fourie (2011) said that few speech-language pathologists have had training in issues related to transference and countertransference and are "often quite unaware of how powerful these forces can be" (p.204). Why do we not learn more effectively from colleagues in psychology how to manage these processes? Possibly because of a traditional lack of confidence in exploring the affective responses that occur during a therapist–client relationship. There is a resistance to exploring these areas of our role. Weld (2012) also notes a fear in supervision in the helping professions of people having emotion-based conversations, perhaps through a fear of not being able to manage what comes forward. There is little training for having these conversations in supervision training, and this may also transfer to conversations within therapy encounters. Without the support of well-trained supervisors, speech and language therapists may avoid the difficult conversations. Geller and Foley (2009) talk about the fact that in the education of speech and language therapists the focus has been more on technical and theoretical knowledge with limited attention paid to exploring the underlying dynamics of clients and families. Luterman (2006) said that "entering the realm of feelings usually strikes fear in the hearts of most speech and hearing professionals because it seems to be out of the scope of practice" (Luterman, 2006, p.9). Geller and Foley (2009) feel that this then leads to resistance or avoidance about looking at affective states and intersubjectivity and how dynamics of relationships influence clinical process. Talking about emotion in supervision is felt to be unsafe territory and certainly in the absence of skilled support and supervision it is.

There needs to be a recognition that we need time to think through emotional responses to what is going on when we are providing therapy, in a supported space. It may be that speech and language therapists are not the best people to provide this. It may be more appropriate for supervision to be provided by, for example, psychology colleagues. Unlike psychotherapists, personal psychotherapy is not considered important in the training of speech and language therapists. The unconscious is given little or no attention.

The lack of acknowledgment of our emotional responses can ultimately lead to a risk of burnout. Ross in Fourie (2011) examines this in more detail, and links the incidence of stress and burnout in the profession and places it within an ecological paradigm, emphasising the fact that the causes of stress and burnout may occur within the work environment rather than within the individual. She says that "in order to promote self-awareness and regulate countertransference responses, practitioners need to have access to skilled supervision… where participants can ventilate and examine feelings… work through concerns and derive emotional support" (p.224). This requires not only skilled supervisors but an acceptance by managers of the need to prioritise the wellbeing of staff, particularly in the face of increasing workloads and reduced resources.

Clearly this has implications for the training of clinical supervisors in the profession. Current provision for clinical supervision training does not necessarily include an examination of these issues. Geller and Foley (2009) propose an alternative way of conceptualising supervision in speech and language therapy. They advocate a framework for training speech and language therapists in supervision which would include skills in focusing on the centrality of relationship at the heart of all learning. Supervisors should be introduced to, and be able to address in supervision, the importance of the therapeutic alliance with supervisees, their use of self, and an ability to discuss internal feeling states that influence the therapeutic relationship, including transference and countertransference. They maintain that for many clinical supervisors the emphasis has been on discipline-specific knowledge, and an adoption of a teaching role within supervision. An emphasis on the concretisation of theoretical knowledge has been at the expense of other types of knowledge, that is, an understanding of the psychodynamic, intrapersonal, subjective, and affective constructs at play during the therapeutic encounter (Geller and Foley, 2009). They go on to say that "the content of most supervision work revolves around the immediate question of 'what to do with the client tomorrow'. Unlike relationship-based practice, the internal, affective, and subjective dimensions of the supervisor–supervisee interactions are less frequently addressed" (p.26).

We have not as a profession embraced the strength of using video in supervision. Video is routinely used in many services to facilitate analysis and discussion of communication difficulties, often in collaboration with parents. It is also used widely in teaching. However, there is little evidence that practising speech and language therapists are routinely using video in supervision. The power of video to support reflective practice is acknowledged but there seems to be a reluctance to use it in supervision. This seems to us to be a missed opportunity. Stokes and Cummins (2013) discuss this reluctance and state that it can be tackled by "a philosophy of supported, systematic, stepped supervision, which is ongoing over time" (p.4). In training on supervision there would be merit in including the videoing of supervision sessions to facilitate deep reflection on body language, styles of language used by the supervisor, and issues that were perhaps touched on but not explored in depth. Hawkins and Shohet (2006) advocate the use of video to review supervision sessions helped by a structured set of questions that have been developed from the work of Kagan (1980). In reviewing a supervision session, the supervisee can be encouraged to think about the following:

1. What did you feel at this point?
2. What were you thinking?
3. What bodily sensations did you have?
4. What did/would you do?
5. What would you have rather done?
6. What problems or risks would there be if you did so?
7. What sort of person does this supervisee see you as?
8. Does this episode remind you of any past situations?
9. Do you have any images or associations in relation to this episode?
10. Are there any other feelings or thoughts that the situation provokes in you?

There is scope to develop this approach within supervision to allow for deeper reflection, assisted by peers or managers. (Hawkins and Shohet, 2006, p.142).

The use of video would support the development of the supervisor by allowing them to become aware of aspects of the session that were not available to them at the time. There is enormous untapped potential in the use of video in supervision practice, as yet unexplored in speech and language therapy supervision.

The increased importance placed on supervision in speech and language therapy is to be welcomed but as a profession we need to guard against it becoming just a part of the bureaucratic process, there to tick the boxes of managing risk, and managerial accountability. There is the potential for supervision to be "a place of learning by both supervisor and supervisee" (Weld, 2012, p.7). She says that supervision should be regarded as a protected learning environment, not a line management surveillance process, and puts the emphasis on partnership, mutual learning, and a sharing of stories. There is a tendency for supervision to focus on the **doing** of therapy rather than the **being** or **becoming** a therapist.

In addition to the use of supervision in examining the affective aspects of the therapeutic relationship, there is scope for supervision to be a place of unpacking and articulating the tacit knowledge that forms the main focus of this book. And yet there is little evidence that this occurs during routine supervision sessions. Supervision has the potential to support speech and language therapists at whatever stage in their careers, to explore the unspoken and unexamined assumptions that underlie professional practice. With skilled supervision, therapists could be encouraged to ask questions such as "What is my rationale for putting a child on review?", "What assumptions am I making about this family's approach to disability in their child?", "How do I know that working on the child's speech sounds using a developmental framework is the right approach?" Supervision is under-used in speech and language therapy as a forum for questioning our received wisdoms. In social work, Munro (2008) talks about how intuitive reasoning can often be the dominant form of decision making. She feels that social workers need time to stop and reflect on what they are doing, and why, in quieter circumstances, outside the daily run of working life. She discusses the fact that emotions may be a valuable source of insight into decision making but it is only through skilled supervision that staff can be made aware of what is influencing their emotional responses. Ryan (2004) says of supervision, "It wakes us up to what we are doing. When we are alive to what we are doing we wake up to what is, instead of falling asleep in the comfort stories of our clinical routines" (p.44). It is all too tempting to rely on the comfort of the clinical routines established in the profession without taking time out to scrutinise and critique them. Effective clinical supervision should be directed at this.

By beginning to explore the potential for an expanded model of supervisory practice, I have drawn attention to some areas that I feel could be more deeply embedded in speech and language therapy supervision. There is such potential in excellent supervision, which can be truly transformative – and has the potential, as Weld (2012) says, of taking exploration of the personal and professional self to a new and exciting level (p.26). Our profession can move supervision away from being a line management surveillance process to a safe protected environment for learning, personal and professional development.

References

ASHA (American Speech-Language Hearing Association) (2008) *Clinical Supervision in Speech-Language Pathology*. Available at http://www.asha.org/policy/TR2008-00296.htm#r50

Bachkirova, T., Jackson, P. & Clutterbuck, D. (2011) *Coaching and Mentoring Supervision Theory and Practice*. Maidenhead: Open University Press.

Bertacchi, J. & Stott, F.M. (1992) A seminar for supervisors in infant/family programs: Growing versus paying more for the same. In E. Fenichel (Ed.) *Learning Through Supervision and Mentorship to Support the Development of Infants, Toddlers and their Families: A Source Book*. Washington, DC: Zero to Three, pp.132–140.

de Shazer, S. (1994) *Words Were Originally Magic*. New York, NY: W.W.Norton.

Dowling, S. (2001) *Supervision: Strategies for Successful Outcomes and Productivity*. Needham Heights, MA: Allyn & Bacon.

Edwards, J.K. (2013) *Strengths-based Supervision in Clinical Practice*. London: Sage Publications.

Ferguson, A. (2008) *Expert Practice: A Critical Discourse*. San Diego: Plural Publishing.

Fourie, R. (2011) (Ed.) *Therapeutic Processes for Communication Disorders*. Hove: Psychology Press.

Geller, E. (2011) Using oneself as a vehicle for change in relational and reflective practice. In R. Fourie (Ed.) *Therapeutic Processes for Communication Disorders*. Hove: Psychology Press, pp.195–212.

Geller, E. & Foley, G. (2009) Broadening the "ports of entry" for speech-language pathologists: A relational and reflective model for clinical supervision. *American Journal of Speech-Language Pathology*, 18, 22–41.

Goolishian, H. (1990) Family therapy: An evolving story. *Contemporary Family Therapy*, 12, 173–180.

Hawkins, P. & Shohet, R. (2012) *Supervision in the Helping Professions*. Maidenhead: Open University Press.

Joshi S. & McAllister, L. (1998) An investigation of supervisory style in speech pathology clinical education. *The Clinical Supervisor*, 17(2), 141–155.

Kadushin, A. (1992) *Supervision in Social Work*. New York: Columbia University Press.

Kagan, N. (1980) Influencing human interaction – eighteen years with IPR. In A.K. Hess (Ed.) *Psychotherapy Supervision: Theory, Research and Practice*. New York: John Wiley & Sons, pp.323–334.

Lubinski R. & Hudson M.W. (2013) *Professional Issues in Speech-Language Pathology and Audiology*. Boston, MA: Delmar Cengage Learning.

Luterman, D.M. (2006) The counseling relationship. *The ASHA Leader*, 11(4), 8–9, 33.

McCluskey, U. (2005) *To Be Met as a Person: The Dynamics of Attachment in Professional Encounters*. London and New York: Karnac.

McCrea, E.S. & Brasseur, J.A. (2003) *The Supervisory Process in Speech-Language Pathology and Audiology*. Boston: Allyn & Bacon.

McDonald, K. (2011) The transference relationship in speech-language therapy. In R. Fourie (Ed.) *Therapeutic Processes for Communication Disorders*. Hove: Psychology Press, pp.169–182.

Milne, D., Sheikh, A., Pattison S. & Wilkinson A. (2011) Evidence-based training for clinical supervisors: A systematic review of 11 controlled studies. *The Clinical Supervisor*, 30(1), 53–71.

Munro, E. (2008) Improving reasoning in supervision. *Social Work Now: The Practice Journal of Child Youth and Family*, 40, 3–9.

Norman-Murch, T. (1996) Reflective supervision as a vehicle for individual and organizational development. *Zero to Three*, October/November, 16–20.

Pearce, P., Phillips, B., Dawson, M. & Leggat, S. (2013) Content of clinical supervision sessions for nurses and allied health professionals: A systematic review. *Clinical Governance*, 18(2), 139–154.

Proctor, B. (2001) Training for the supervision alliance attitude, skills and intention. In J.R. Cutcliffe, T. Butterworth & B. Proctor *Fundamental Themes in Clinical Supervision*. London. Routledge, pp.25–46.

RCSLT (2012) Supervision guidelines for speech and language therapists. www.rcslt.org

Ross, E. (2011) Burnout and self-care in the practice of speech pathology and audiology: An ecological perspective. In R. Fourie (Ed.) *Therapeutic Processes for Communication Disorders*. Hove: Psychology Press, pp.213–228.

Ryan, S. (2004) *Vital Practice*. Portland, UK: Sea Change Publications.

Seligman, M.E.P. & Csikszentmihalyi, M. (2000) Positive psychology: An introduction. *American Psychologist*, 55(1), 5–14.

Silverman, E-M. (2011) Self-reflection in clinical practice. In R. Fourie (Ed.) *Therapeutic Processes for Communication Disorders*. Hove: Psychology Press, pp.183–193.

Simpson, S & Sparkes, C. (2008) Are you getting enough? Speech and language therapy in practice. Available from http://www.scribd.com/doc/142737673/Are-you-getting-enough-1-Supervision-in-context

Sparkes, C & Simpson, S (2013) Supporting robust supervision practice. *Bulletin*, 730, Feb 2013, 22–23.

Spence, S., Wilson, J., Kavanagh, D., Strong, J. & Worrall, L. (2001) Clinical supervision in four mental health professions: A review of the evidence. *Behavior Change*, 18, 135–155.

Stokes, J. & Cummins, K. (2013) Video use in reflective practice: Experience from educating speech and language therapists. *Compass: Journal of Learning and Teaching*, 4(7). Available at https://journals.gre.ac.uk/index.php/compass/article/view/82

Stoltenberg, C. & Delworth, U. (1987) *Supervising Counselors and Therapists: A Developmental Approach*. San Francisco: Jossey-Bass Wiley.

Walsh, F. (2006) *Strengthening Family Resiliency*. New York, NY: Guilford Press.

Weld, N. (2012) *A Practical Guide to Transformative Supervision for the Helping Professions: Amplifying Insight*. London: Jessica Kingsley.

White, M. & Epston, D. (1990) *Narrative Means to Therapeutic Ends*. New York, NY: W.W. Norton.

4 Using video to catch, develop and propagate emerging skills with parents, children, educators and therapists

Keena Cummins

Within speech and language therapy practice with children there are a range of different approaches. The most common scenario involves the following: a child is identified as having a problem, the child is referred to a therapist. The therapist assesses the child's strengths and areas for development through a range of structured formal and informal assessments. On the basis of this a choice of different therapy approaches is on offer. Some of them are versions of the expert model: the therapist works with the parent to address the area of difficulty through a range of different approaches but remains in control and is directing the process based on his or her greater understanding of communication difficulties. Some of these approaches are more collaborative, placing the family at the centre. Some of them are an amalgam of the two. The majority focus on the presenting 'diagnosis' of the child.

One of the approaches which has developed over the last 30 years is working through video and interaction in order to support children presenting with communication difficulties. This chapter explores the strengths of this approach and gives the rationale for its use, drawing on the literature on attachment and interaction development in children. I argue that all speech and language therapy should be based on these principles from the outset: video use, parents at the centre and adult self-reflection. We should place parents at the heart of our practice and video provides us with the necessary opportunity for our own continuous, ongoing professional self-reflection. The particular approach that I have developed uses aspects of the collaborative model of therapy but goes further in the partnership that it fosters between child, parent and therapist. The term 'parents' acknowledges the wide range of people who might be in a parental role in children's lives.

Twenty years ago I inherited the phenomenal model of parent–child interaction therapy (Kelman and Schneider, 1994), which at the time of my inheritance consisted of weekly parent workshops, children's groups and individual video sessions over six weeks. It was offered through an impairment-based model of service delivery to one 'type' of presenting communication difficulty, i.e., those children who presented with severe language delay and specific language impairment and to those parents who were perceived to need 'support' in their parenting skills. Within weeks I had met Sonia who I believe changed my whole concept of the role of speech and language therapy. On the first day, Sonia watched herself on screen at play with her son and noticed how much she was chatting. She did not notice how skilled she was in every other way and sadly nor had many other people (she had left school early, was currently on medication for depression and was perceived by many early years health care professionals as challenging and difficult). I did not need to teach her anything; what I did need to do was be clearly analytical in my own mind about the many skills that she had (which at a superficial level were being masked by her questioning and domination of the interaction) and to wait and see what was visible to her when she looked at herself and her child on the screen. She immediately saw just how much she was talking (compensating) and wondered what would happen if she stopped asking questions. She played with her son again offering silence and her little boy started to initiate more. I fed in some theory and asked that she carry on experimenting in this way for five minutes a day. I waited the week to see what the outcome would be. I was blown away. In a week Ron had gone from fleeting attention and single words to focused attention and three-word phrases. He had previously received three months of 1:1 therapy with a therapist without the parent present, who perceived him as having learning difficulties and had referred him for a child development team assessment. Sonia did not need workshops, her child did not need children's groups. What she, like all other parents and indeed we ourselves needed, was to be respected in her significant role, listened to and understood, appreciated for her personality and knowledge and offered the opportunity to reflect with support on her child's interaction timing and her responses. Having seen herself in action Sonia relished the chance to experiment and explore with what she had just learnt about the theory behind her behaviours and then to watch it back to see if her adapted behavior had an impact on her son. When it did she could not wait to try it at home, fine-tuning our discussion to blend with the family's own set-up. What Ron needed was for the therapist to respect that the most skilled person (his mother) was the one continuing to support his emerging skills.

Sonia confirmed my belief that the only way to start working with children with communication difficulties is with their parents as **research partners** through video. Consequently, we developed an approach to service delivery which ensured that all parents received a course of video therapy on accessing the service (Cummins and Hulme, 2001) with their child's potential 'diagnosis' being irrelevant to their access.

There are lessons to be learned from the particular style of relationship building that arises from working through video which is supported by the research underpinning interaction. It is the focus on reflective practice, attunement through regulation and body watching in parents and their children which emerges from video use, that can teach us so much as a profession in every area of our work. In the early days, my reading was mostly specific to speech and language therapy, but over the years I have had the luxury of accessing extensive research and theory across a wide range of different professional groups which has compounded my understanding of why certain elements of interaction are so fundamental to communication development. The most enjoyable and biggest learning opportunity for myself has of course been the opportunity to work extensively with families from a wide range of cultures and socio-economic groups in different areas of the UK, who have eagerly reflected on their abilities and individual circumstances and provided empirical evidence of their own impact.

Video use has provided me with a mirror to hold up to the profession. Through its constant use with families, speech and language therapists, student speech and language therapists and educators, I have come to realise the power of video to challenge the way we traditionally manage and provide services. This has led me to seriously doubt the effectiveness of many other models of working. In this chapter, I outline the approach that I have continued to develop, detailing what we can learn from video, giving rationales for the use of video therapy and outlining some basic principles of the work I believe to be most effective.

What video has taught us

Over the last 50 years there has been an explosion in our understanding of human development, relationships, interaction and how we learn. Central to this understanding has been the development of technology and video, bringing the opportunity to analyse in minute detail with freeze frame the tiny signals that we provide, read, interpret and respond to whenever we engage with another person. It is now possible to unpick the minutiae of significant behaviours in individuals and to observe their impact on another person's confidence, communication and language. We can identify the cause, effect and feedback loop of interaction and integrate what families tell us from their knowledge and perspective with what we know from our experience. As the psychotherapist Sue Gerhardt states, we have also hit an exciting time where we have "begun to integrate disciplines that have for far too long been kept in rigid compartments" (Gerhardt, 2005, p.5). We have started to "communicate and influence each other" (p.2) and identify key components in emotional development, attachment, communication, interaction, learning and identity that are not only profoundly important for 'clients' of all ages and presenting communication difficulties but are highly significant for ourselves personally and are key to the role of us as a profession. This consilience (Wilson, 1998, p.1) or unity of knowledge of common findings between disciplines is reshaping our concept of therapy.

The importance of understanding attachment, synchrony and relationships

Bowlby's seminal attachment theory (1969), complemented by Ainsworth and Bell (1970) and Ainsworth et al.'s (1978) description of patterns of attachment, specified the essential ingredients of the initial relationships between babies and their 'primary care givers' (usually parents). They defined how significant those patterns are in the development of self-confidence and access to opportunities both in the developing infant and consequently throughout life. Through frame-by-frame analysis using video, Stern (1985) identified the 'attunement' of parents as being fundamental to supporting the child in calming itself and learning to self-regulate. The parent attunes or mirrors the child's feelings momentarily (e.g., if the child is tearful the parent's face will momentarily mirror a sad expression) and then purposefully misattunes, (modelling a soothing expression). This shows empathy for how the child is feeling whilst supporting the child in self-calming and moving out of their over-stimulated state. From this secure and calm state the baby is able to experiment and explore and learn. The parent provides "timely adaptation to distress and social cues" (Feldman, 2007, p.331). As the infant grows older, they become increasingly able to regulate themselves both when a parent is present and when they are not. Caregivers' responses lead to the development of patterns of attachment and internal working models (or habits of behaviours, interaction and learning styles), which influence each individual's perceptions, emotions, thoughts and expectations in later relationships and throughout life (Bretherton and Munholland, 1999; Heard, Lake and McCluskey, 2009; McCluskey, 2005).

Although temperaments always differ – some babies "may be born more reactive and sensitive to stimulation than others" (Gerhardt, 2005, p.20) – it is the consistent attunement of the parent that supports each child in becoming robust and resilient, regardless of their nature.

Through video, researchers have been able to see just how balanced and actively involved the developing infant is, and how bidirectional or 'intersubjective' parent–child relationships are (see Beebe et al. (2003) for a detailed summary of the theory of intersubjectivity). The child influences the parent and vice versa, the infant and adult mirroring one another's expressions in "a delicate and immediate with-the-other awareness" (Trevarthen, 1993, p.122) that forms the basis of all communication before words. Child and parent regulate one another in their "intricate rhythmic patterns" (Trevarthen and Aitken, 2001, p.5) of interaction that is predominantly non-verbal, a two-way sharing of control which is specific to individual cultures and underpins all developing language. These fundamental non-verbal behaviours, defined by Bateson (1975) as protoconversation, consist of focused attention (face watching), mirroring of one another, taking turns, longer pauses, higher pitch, facial expression and hand gestures.

It is this success in synchrony, 'balance of control' and uniqueness in interaction that supports the child in perceiving themselves as equal and significant and gives them the confidence to establish, explore and maintain relationships and opportunities within other contexts and with other people. Through experimentation, trial and error and the immediate response of others, the child co-constructs his or her communication, experiences and 'vitality' (McCluskey, 2005). The child develops an ability to influence others and the environment whilst still turning to the "caregiver to provide him with information about the nature of the world, internal and external" (Fonagy, Gergely and Target, 2007, p.312).

The relevance of synchrony in understanding communication difficulties

It is understood that children with communication difficulties give off weaker communication signals or have difficulties in these signals being read because their initiations are not as rapid, consistent, clear, efficient or as effective as their peers. As Roberts and Kaiser (2011) suggest, they may "differ from typical children in rate of communication, development of joint attention (Mundy et al., 1995), clarity of communicative intention, intelligibility (Rice, Sell and Hadley, 1991), and responsiveness to language (Wetherby, Prizant and Hutchinson, 1998)" (p.181). Indeed, "children whose speech cannot be understood are less likely to elicit language-facilitating interactions from significant others" (Yoder, Camarata and Gardner, 2005, p.34). "Children with communication difficulties might use roughly the same skill set, but not be as efficient or effective as typical learners" (Alt, Meyers and Ancharski, 2012, p.491). This makes it hard for parents, adults and friends to know how to respond, and influences the synchrony of interaction and the subtle elements in their attachment systems. The mutual balance and regulatory or calming patterns between the child, parent and others become mismatched. This can be perceived by the adult as a sign of attention or behavioural difficulties in the child. This then affects how the partnership is able to build ideas together.

As the child appears to do less, so the communicative partners start to overcompensate and increase in directiveness, i.e., to take responsibility for the interaction. This in turn affects the child's opportunity and reason for communicating, and particularly influences their use of eye contact. The synchrony of interaction becomes increasingly discordant and the child settles into a passive, disengaged or confrontational role in attempting to contribute or manage the situation.

The confidence of both the parent and child becomes negatively affected and the parent through anxiety becomes focused on what they feel they have omitted to do and what they perceive their child to be unable to do. The parent and child do not have attachment issues per se, but the synchrony of attunement and attachment is affected.

Focused individualised video interaction therapy

There are currently interactionalist models of therapy with a growing evidence base: Intensive Interaction (Nind and Hewett, 2005), SCERTS model (Prizant et al., 2006), Hanen (www.hanen.org) and Relationship Development Intervention (Gutstein, 2009). These have had a profound impact on our profession. The premise of these approaches is to support parents and adults in generally reflecting on their timing of interaction in order to support the child's underlying self-regulation and confidence and competence as a communicator, whilst adapting the environment and optimising visual support. Models of video interaction include the Michael Palin parent–child interaction model (Botterill and Kelman, 2009) and the Video Interaction Guidance (VIG) model that over a 4–6 week period supports parental attunement through video playback (Kennedy, Landor and Todd, 2011). In this approach, clinicians have successfully addressed the needs of a "range of clients and contexts, including infants, vulnerable families, schools, children and adults on the autistic continuum and children with hearing impairment" (Kennedy et al., 2011, p.16).

Parents as a fulcrum

I would advocate that optimum impact is achieved when the parents at the outset are seen as the fulcrum to therapy through individualised video support. Therapy has to be done via parents. The relationship with the parent and how the parent feels about themselves defines the outcome of therapy. By recognising the parents as the fulcrum to interaction, language and learning we optimise their skill and ensure that they are the hinge to enhancing therapeutic impact and reaching the core of the child's developing system, offering optimum therapy in a relatively short space of time. Self-regulation and the synchrony of mutual attunement, and space for silence form the basis for the system of all communicative intent, language development, speech sound development and fluency. "The synchronizing caregiver thus facilitates the infant's information processing by adjusting the mode, amount, variability, and timing of the onset and offset of stimulation to the infant's actual integrative capacities" (Schore, 2001, p.19). Ensuring that the synchrony of the relationship is re-established is fundamental.

Parent–child attachment (and consequent support of self-regulation and reading and influencing communication) is central to the development of this system which is "circular not linear" (Gerhardt, 2004, p.9). As Schore (2001) stresses, the process is psychoneurobiological, every element impacting on every other element: autonomic, limbic, biological, neurological, psychological, environmental and cultural. The interpersonal environment positively affects the experience-dependent developing brain. "Interactions with the environment especially relationships with other people, directly shape the development of the brain's structure and function" (Siegel, 2012, p.xiv). Recent brain scanning techniques have provided evidence of neurons and biochemical reactions in the brain that are being triggered rapidly by all stimuli and are laying down connections, feedback loops which are continuously firing, interlinking and weaving complex neural maps which are affected by repetition, habit and reinforcement. These maps can be re-patterned and reinforced due to the neuroplasticity of the brain (Doidge, 2007).

Through video, the parent becomes familiar with the patterns of their child's communication and re-patterns the balance in their interaction and the consequent neural pathways. The synchrony re-establishes, the parent knows how to react and respond, and the child and parent self-propagate change with increasingly less dependency on the therapist. "Once a pattern of attuned interactions is established or re-established, an attuned relationship develops which reaches well beyond simple interaction patterns to form new emotions and identities" (Kennedy et al., 2011, p.22).

Common misperceptions

A common misperception concerning parental involvement in speech and language therapy is that only certain 'types' of parent need to 'learn interaction' or that only certain types of presenting communication difficulty are appropriate for video therapy, or that there is a certain 'age' or 'stage' at which interaction therapy and video therapy are relevant. This is indicative of a clear misunderstanding of the complexity and bidirectional nature of interaction, recent research developments in language, communication, learning development and plasticity of the brain. Intuitive interaction occurs in all parent–child relationships and is not related to academic background, socio-economic or sociocultural experience. The parent comes to speech and language therapy with life experience that in many areas exceeds that of the therapist. The exchange of such experience is complementary, informative and a necessity. The video is not a means to show someone how to interact but is a means of exploration for both therapist and parent in order to understand the emerging skills of each child and optimum ways of supporting them in accessing the child's ongoing opportunities and limitless potential. It is a fully engaging collaboration.

Why use parent video reflection from the outset?

By watching any child's interaction back on a screen, the adults are able to analyse the child's skills and consequently explore behaviours in themselves that optimally support the child. Video focuses on the interaction timing of the parent and child and the characteristics of the child's emerging communication skills. The video is a means of providing an objective visual and auditory image of the child's signals, which are often so subtle that they will be missed without the use of playback. It should be a necessary requirement of any 'assessment' or 'observation' of a child. It provides opportunities to observe reliably the child's self regulation, play patterns, eye contact and face watching, attention and listening skills, communicative intent, language and speech abilities whilst looking at the impact these have on the adult. Simultaneously, it offers the opportunity to analyse what enhances those skills and what may inhibit. Whatever the level of communication difficulty or the cause behind it, the priority of therapy is to make the parent and child feel capable, valued and vital and in so doing to observe the spontaneous skills evolve within the family relationship through patterning successful signals and responses.

The use of video as a therapeutic intervention

Video therapy is not 'training', a 'course' or a 'programme'. It is a process of therapeutic intervention. It needs to be carried out individually for optimum efficacy and takes place over a period of a minimum of four consecutive weeks in order to ensure consistency, reinforcement and patterning of clear signals. The synchrony of interaction is rapid and complex. Video makes explicit significant elements that are often 'concealed' in everyday life. In focusing on the detail with the intensity of the freeze frame and playback, specific behaviours are seen and intensified for the observers. It provides time and space for the parent and therapist to explore this detail and supports the adult in focusing and reinforcing the child's less resilient characteristics in order to make them stronger.

Children with communication difficulties do not differ from their peers who are "active participants who learn to affect the behavior and attitudes of others through active signaling and who gradually learn to use more sophisticated and conventional means to communicate through caregivers' contingent social responsiveness" (Dunst, Lowe and Bartholomew, 1990, p.40). Children with communication difficulties have not as yet learned how to positively affect the behaviour and attitude of others. By taking time to support the child in active signalling, the synchrony of more conventional means is re-established and language is scaffolded through labelling, recasting and extending. Through video the parent is shown how they are using each skill identified as supportive in interaction development. At the start of the process, their child cannot maintain synchrony at the pace at which those skills are being presented. So, for a period of time (usually over a month) these skills in the adult are stripped down in order to make each one salient and clear for the child. As the weeks progress, and the child becomes more robust in their signals, so the parent gradually reintroduces other skills commensurate with the pace of acquisition and development of the child. What appears to be a slow process in the first few weeks, propagates and increases in pace as the child assimilates and uses each skill confidently. The child's engine for communication becomes increasingly active and faster. The process starts by making the underlying fundamental non-verbal behaviours robust. As the child and parent become increasingly confident in their experimentation and spontaneity so they become more autonomous and independent, the parent being able to reflect back and discuss each area of skill confidently. As they do so, their confidence in influencing other situations and experimenting with their own ideas becomes increasingly evident. By the parent fully understanding and experiencing the significant means by which the child seeks and scaffolds their communication and language, the parent is then confident to support the child's ongoing experience. In focusing on the strengths and emerging skills, the less constructive behaviours diminish and the parent becomes enthused and captivated by the child's spontaneity and uniqueness, starting to enjoy the creativity of their relationship rather than worrying about the things they are not doing. As the child becomes reinforced intrinsically through their enjoyment of what they are doing and the positive responses and reinforcement they receive, so they increase their desire to court more positive interactions. This has a profound impact on those children who may initially have presented as having behavioural difficulties.

The key elements to the process of video support are:

- Sessions are held individually with the family.

- The parent/s are filmed interacting with their child in a way that is most comfortable for the dyad and in which they are having fun.

- They are given time to watch that interaction on screen and note whatever they wish to.

- The parents are supported in observing (through a therapist-facilitated observation sheet) the strategies that they are using intuitively that research has proven effective in supporting interaction and communication development. The video is not edited. Parents are very able to watch successful moments and their impact finding the contrast of less successful moments useful.

- The therapist clarifies why these particular elements of interaction are so fundamental to the process of evolving communication, language and learning.

- The parents then hypothesise which particular strategy may be having the most positive effect and they are re-filmed interacting with their child once more optimising that one strategy (which makes it salient for the child) then and there.

- Therapist and parents watch the updated video and assess the immediate impact on the child of the salient strategy. Having assessed the success of its implementation the parent applies that strategy for five minutes daily at home whilst the child is doing something they enjoy. This can be indoors, outside, material-focused or during interactive games.

- Consistency and daily implementation of just one element is essential in order to pattern/map the behaviour both in the adult and the child.

- The following week the parents report back their experiences, explaining what worked best for them within their context and raising questions pertinent to their application and the child's developing skills.

- A new video is taken from which the therapist is able to provide theory and observations matched to the understanding and behaviours of the parent and child targeting their specific needs at that moment in time. If at this point it is appropriate for the parents to build on another strategy (which has often been developed intuitively responding to their child's emerging skills) then this is focused on.

- Each session builds on the previous session at the child's rate of emergence.

Through individualised video the therapist can ensure that the concepts being worked with are specific to the child and parent at the moment they are needed. Questions and answers reflect the detail of the child and the enquiry of the parent. Understanding and application are experimented with there and then and the hypothesis of the therapist tested. There is little room for misunderstanding. The reflection is fine-tuned and in no way general or superfluous. The session goes straight to the point and is therefore specific and efficient in terms of time and resources. It is essential that no one is overloaded. Therapy 'holds' the parent and gives them 'time' to explore what is salient for them and their child, whilst giving the therapist time to learn what is important and of value to the family and their child's emerging skills. The vocabulary and language used become highly meaningful as it is watched in action and a 'shared vocabulary' becomes established. The child is never pulled or pushed but is supported through their 'zone of proximal development', (Vygotsky, 1962, 1978), i.e., the gap between what a child can do alone and what they can do with the help of someone more skilled or experienced, adult or child within play and communicatively. The child gradually re-organises their systematisation of communicative signals and increases their confidence in experimentation. Parent and therapist have pleasure in seeing the specific developments of each child week on week, the outcomes being clearly evident on film.

The younger the child is, the easier patterning or re-patterning is likely to be, but regardless of the age of the child (I have worked with children up to 15 years of age), focusing on the synchrony of interaction for a course of video therapy has a marked impact on the child's communication and learning abilities. "Change is possible; neurogenesis and neuroplasticity – the creation of new neurons and new neuronal connections continue throughout our life spans. Experience alters the brain, even as we age" (Fishbane, 2007, p.397). The child, parent and therapist develop together at a pace pertinent for the child.

Video challenges our own perceptions and frameworks. Supporting a parent in focusing on a particular element and leaving them to experiment and explore with it over the week leads to emerging skills that are unique to the child and parent, shifting the expectations of the therapist and challenging any subjectivity or preconceived ideas. The nature of the relationship between parent and therapist becomes similar to that of 'supervision', i.e., to support the parent in exploring and monitoring their own abilities and their impact in order to empower the child optimally. There is little difference in the way that video interaction is used to support parents or professionals (e.g., speech and language therapists, educators). As adults we are all students in the child's developing interaction, the video is a means of seeing and analysing that interaction. We are interdependent.

Video therapy is often carried out in the family's first language with the parent interpreting for the therapist, or through an interpreter. The principles are the same. The parent becomes highly mindful of specific elements of their own interaction skills being able to self-monitor their own input on an ongoing basis. The therapist manages the session, the system and the consistency, and offers support and discussion to complement the parents' emerging awareness and theory base.

Video is a starting point, a means for discussion and the quickest way to re-establish the foundations of communication from which the child and parent can self-propagate. It is a means of joint understanding between parent and therapist and other professionals all of whom become students of each child's emerging interaction. The primary axis of change remains the parent.

Specific technological advances have shifted in that we now have many domestic experiences on video on i-Pads, telephones etc. – evidence of people in a relaxed environment doing what they like to do in the way their family normally carries out their routines. This provides us with true insight into the family. We have no excuses for carrying out therapy that does not optimise these opportunities.

Key principles involved in optimal support of parents

Personalisation. Each one of us perceives and interprets things differently. Successful therapy is based on the relationship that the therapist builds with the parent right from the outset. This relationship is based on attunement, body watching, feedback, repair and mirroring (see later). The video supports this relationship by ensuring that the therapist and parent understand each other's meaning and perspective by seeing it in action on the screen. This ensures that accompanying theory used can be developed and matched in line with the parent's current knowledge and understanding and practice in a way that makes sense at the time that it is needed.

A **joint vocabulary** is truly established which optimises the sociocultural beliefs and values of each family. By providing individual time the therapist is able to observe and listen to the concerns, vulnerabilities and skills of each individual and then provide information that complements the individuals' understanding whilst observing how that information is interpreted and applied.

Independence. Parents become increasingly confident in managing and influencing their child's development and in observing and understanding other environments, supporting others in reflecting on their timing when communicating with their child and becoming increasingly confident in experimenting and exploring their own ideas and creativity. As the parent and child's synchrony re-establishes, so their autonomy increases. They are able to express the progress their child has made, specify where their child is at and identify what supports their child. They become more confident in making informed decisions about their child's future needs if they continue to be related to their communication and learning abilities. They are also in a position to provide video evidence of their child's communication skills over time and the strategies that best support them providing a visual focus for meetings around the child that can shape and consolidate the focus of professional advice.

Key points of focus in video therapy

Over the years, as my understanding and my experience of working with parents and children have deepened, I have become increasingly aware of just how important eye contact and face watching are and how formative they are in underpinning all relationships.

Silence, eye contact and face watching

If the child is going to hold an influence on others and be confident in their influence, it needs to be on their own terms in their own time, when they choose to initiate and at the rate at which they initiate. Children with communication difficulties may well be engaging in eye contact but their **influence** through eye contact has lost its impact and meaning. This is only evident through video, within which it is possible to show the distinction between a child looking and a child influencing with their eyes. When a child is robust in their communication they trigger the adult's response through looking at the adult and initiating through pointing or vocalising. More importantly, when they look away the adult knows to stop, to become silent. The adult attending to this signal is essential to the child's sense of control in communication and in their ability to self-regulate, self-calm and turn-take. The child "will turn away in an effort to regulate the release of chemicals flowing through his body" (Banks, 2011, p.174). Overstimulation leads to anxiety and the release of the anxiety hormone cortisol. When an adult is concerned about a child's ability they can become intrusive, and the child will manage as best they can, i.e., avoid eye contact providing themselves with physiological relief (Heard et al., 2009, p.87). As Stern (2002) notes, the adult needs to watch the child's face and gaze aversion as a cue to lower the level of their own adult behaviour. As adults, we often misconstrue children's 'lack' of eye contact. We perceive not looking as being negative rather than as a positive indicator of how we should behave. This often results in misleading advice such as using alerters (e.g., name or touch), which I would argue merely compounds a child's passivity in the relationship through adult control. Respecting the child looking away as a signal for the adult to stop talking is essential. Waiting for the eye contact signal before saying a word shows the adult when the child is ready and starts the process of shared attention. When the child does look up the parent either smiles or says a word which releases beta-endorphin and dopamine (feel-good hormones) (Schore, 2003) and the parent and child automatically mirror each other's facial expression. Engaging in eye contact triggers the mutual release of the opiate oxytocin (Fonagy, Gergely and Target, 2007). Schore notes (2001) that we understand how another person is feeling from their facial expressions without conscious awareness and that we innately mirror one another's behaviours. It has been suggested that this mirroring of actions and emotions of others affects the neuronal processing in our brains (Gallese, Keysers and Rizzolatti, 2004) and that it is this mirroring that is fundamental in mutual understanding, interaction (Ramachandran, 2011), understanding emotions and developing a vocabulary.

Silence, self-regulation and exploration

By the adult waiting for the child to choose to look, by being in their personal space (the listening space that indicates the adult is ready to respond), silent and interested in what they are doing, the adult allows the child time to self-regulate, to calm themselves, to coordinate their action (gross and fine motor), to focus on something they are enjoying doing, and to experiment and explore without any pressure to communicate. Silence is a strong form of stimulation. The child "focusing through play and interaction learns both emotional and cognitive self-regulation" (Florez, 2011, p.47). The child learns to regulate thoughts, emotions and behaviours, which in turn helps them to engage in and enjoy challenging learning activities. The child may move away but as the adult remains rooted at the activity the child will return and re-engage. Their attention and concentration development (Cooper, Modley and Reynell, 1978) increases. So too does their understanding of cause and effect, trial and error and 'complexity' of play and their comfort in non-verbal extension of their play ideas. Fundamental to the adult's understanding is how 'stimulating' silence is, that in the adult remaining silent (until asked by the child's eyes to comment or respond) the child has time to think and do. The child is the engine. The parent starts to enjoy the activity and it becomes a pleasure rather than a 'task'. The child learns how to court the adult's response through calm exploration, eye contact and turn-taking. Behaviour that may previously have been perceived as difficult starts to settle as the child learns the influence of their ideas. The child becomes intrinsically motivated (Brown, 2007), the pleasure of the task, the interaction and the relationship being in themselves enjoyable and rewarding. As a consequence, what Molden and Dweck (2006) describe as the child's 'learning self-identity' develops. This is their belief that they can learn and change themselves. Miller and Stiver (1997) suggest that good connection leads to a desire for more good connections as the adult waits and watches, only speaking when the child looks up. Eye contact and face watching become literally addictive (because of the mutual opiates exchanged) so the child visibly 'patterns' to the success of the outcomes of controlling the adult's contributions with their eyes. Most importantly, the adult learns just when to offer information and when to stop and offer processing time (silence). As the weeks progress, so do the child's abilities in self-regulation, attention, exploration, experimentation, face watching, emotion reading and lip reading. They also learn the benefit of taking time in silence to think and organise themselves, time to integrate their skills and synthesise information.

Development of vocabulary and sentence structure through naming, repeating, recasting and extending

Once the child starts to look and vocalise, parents will naturally recast and extend their child's utterances. A recast, as described by Saxton (2005), is where a more experienced speaker responds to what a child says by expanding, deleting, or changing their utterances while maintaining the meaning. This supports the child in hearing how close their word or sentence is to the accurate one, and this leads to a re-attempt with success the next time. The adult naturally supports the element that is currently vulnerable, e.g., stressing difficult speech sounds (Camarata, Nelson and Camarata, 1994). If it is grammar, the adult responds by stressing grammatical markers, making them salient and clear for the child and supporting the child's repair.

Repair and persistence

As the child develops in their face watching so they learn to watch the adult's reaction or to monitor the response of the other person and repair any breakdowns in communication. Wetherby and Prizant (1996) define repair as being the ability to persist in communication and to modify or revise a signal when faced with a breakdown in communication. Opportunities for repair are offered when attempts are not responded to as intended. Holler and Wilkin (2011) point out that in interacting, people create meaning jointly, through what has been referred to as an iterative process, with the aim of establishing mutual understanding. This collaborative process has been referred to as grounding (Clark and Brennan 1991). Grounding leads to synchronisation between the partners involved, "on various levels, including wording, syntax, speaking rate, gestures, eye-gaze fixations, body position, postural and sometimes pronunciation" (Brennan, Galati and Kuhle, 2010, p. 306). It is frequently far from perfect and involves each partner watching the other closely repairing any breakdowns through repetition and re-clarification. Each person says something and monitors the other's reaction to see if any repair or augmentation is required. General dialogue is full of false starts, ill formed utterances and misperceptions.

In the early stages of video therapy, when the adult is experimenting with silence, the child may vocalise or point but not look at the adult. In so doing they are not providing opportunity for feedback, grounding and repair. If the parent answers the child without waiting for the child to look up first, they are compounding the child's pattern of talking without looking. The parent is therefore encouraged not to respond until the child looks at them. If the adult remains silent, the child will keep repeating and then finally look to gain a response. The adult speaks only when and as soon as the child looks up.

Within therapy this can feel unresponsive, but the child quickly realises that they need to look to the parent's face for a verbal and non-verbal response. The face watching pattern is relatively quickly patterned if the parent remains consistent. In so doing, the adult lets the child take responsibility for repair and supports them in watching for feedback. Emotion reading and mirroring become integral to the process of grounding. This also supports a child who is unclear in their speech and is patterned to face watch through the adult's repetition. The adult is able to repeat intelligible speech because they have understood it but unable to repeat unintelligible speech which will show as confusion on their face. The child will read that the adult has not understood and will repeat with increased clarity. By waiting for the child to look up we are also supporting mutual lip reading which makes clarity easier. The child repairs by looking at the adult and repeating again, usually with a closer approximation which leads to the adult understanding and saying the word in the mature form (phonological recasting).

By working on this visual bi-directional feedback we are supporting each child in becoming attuned to the subtle signals that we elicit as co-communicators, supporting them in being responsible within the dialogue and providing the child with recasts that support their developing language system. Therapy remains the same whether communication, language or speech, i.e., face watching, feedback, repair and co-construction and supportive recasting at the level of the child's current difficulty.

Resilience and independence

Demos (1989) defines resilience as being the ability to move within an interaction and relationship from a positive effect to a negative effect and back to the positive. It is directly related to repair. With each successful repair that the child makes they are becoming more resilient, confident to trial something and adapt it accordingly. In supporting a parent through the process of re-synchronisation of their child's interaction and waiting for their child's eye contact/facewatching, the adult becomes contingent with what the child wants to express rather than guessing. The child becomes confident in their ability to manage themselves and others through watching, initiating, engaging, listening, verbalising, responding and repairing. They start to experiment with and receive positive reinforcement from an increasing number of adults and peers with whom they mutually provide recasts and extensions. They also start to manage the rate of their communicative partner. This has a direct impact on their confidence, self-esteem, language, communication, social skills and learning development. They perceive themselves as a significant engine in the interaction. Their signals become accurately perceived and others engage with them naturally (without feeling anxiety) on an equal footing. The concentric circles of reinforcement from everyone in the child's environment spontaneously develop.

The child feels increasingly vital and confident. The adult shows/models how to truly listen. For the majority of children and their parents, once this process has been established no further intervention is required. The parent has been the agent of change, they know what they are doing and why, are adaptive, reflective and skilled and, most importantly are confident in exactly what they do naturally to support their child's ongoing process. For those children with more complex needs, further support is offered through video, focusing on visual support, augmentative support and environmental adaptation at home and within an educational context.

How we learn from this approach

In my experience, no other forms of therapy offer the same rate of change in the client or the same opportunities to mediate skills and fully optimise collaborative contributions as individualised video. Scaffolding theory on to the innate skills of the parent is far more efficient than any modelling, explaining, presenting, facilitating or role-playing. Given the opportunity to positively reflect on yourself in action and to be responsible for the marked change in your own child has a discernible impact on adult self-esteem which in turn leads to the child's self-confidence, joint exploration, experimentation, trial, error, enjoyment and independence.

Video interaction within an educational context

Experience of working in this way has led me to question what we perceive to be the priority and order of things in speech and language therapy. Over the past decade I have been working in nursery settings and schools (primary and secondary) through video interaction using the same model as with parents in order to support the staff that know the child best and who work with them daily. The staff bring videos of themselves and the child carrying out tasks they are required to do (e.g., play activities in the early years, from the curriculum in the older years) and the staff through video reflect collaboratively with the speech and language therapist on their own interaction skills and their impact on the child's learning and communication development.

Nind and Hewett (2005) have identified some key aspects of interaction that are vulnerable to erosion with educationalists when working with children with communication difficulties and/or learning needs. These parallel the overcompensation strategies common to parents such as difficulty in seeing intentionality and signals, reduced pauses, reduced celebration of behaviours and adult dominance. There has also been much written about the connection between communication difficulties and perceived primary or secondary behaviour difficulties and mental health (Durkin and Conti-Ramsden, 2010). An interactionalist perspective recognises that each element influences the others and that developing the child's self-regulation and face watching will pattern positive behaviour and develop the child's communication skills, learning self-identity, learning independence, resilience and autonomy. Molden and Dweck (2006) have noted that those children with a learning self-identity, regardless of their tested intelligence, are more successful in school than those with a fixed identity and are more confident in how they relate to others. The child's self-confidence increases because "judgements of significant others are incorporated over time into one's own self–concept" (Caldwell et al., 2004, p.1142).

In working within schools through video our profession deepens its understanding of the demands of the curriculum on both the child and the adults. Time and money are invested in effecting positive change with individual children whilst engaging the practitioners in active reflective learning which they are then in a position to generalise and apply to other children. The child's skills and evolving abilities are catalogued on video and are shared with the other practitioners and professionals, e.g., in case reviews or in moving up to the next year group, providing evidence of specific strategies of support. In this way, we remain learner-centred and child-specific, and work within the organisational structure, interfacing communication difficulties with curriculum demands and continuity of academic course work. This enables inclusion and provides effective management through congruency, consistency, predictability and reliability within and between adults regardless of their profession.

We now have clear evidence that interaction, communication and learning are interdependent and bi-directional and that targeting the child's emerging skills and learning self-identity effects most change.

I have grave concerns about many care pathways for school-aged children, which entail an advisory service or a model of service delivery that segregates communication from learning. Assessing the child from a purely communicative, linguistic or phonological perspective by a speech and language therapist through observation sheets in class and in isolation is inadequate. Writing lengthy reports from this unrepresentative information is time-consuming and provides static information about a child. Targets are given which frequently focus on the language 'problem' capping the child's opportunity and potential by making the adult focus on goals that frequently do not take into account emerging skills. This may lead to signals of vitality being inadvertently missed. Holding lengthy meetings around the child with advice from many external professionals generally overwhelms the education practitioner who is actually working with the child and frequently does not take into account the successful skills they are already using. The cost of such a model is high. There may be a place for formal, dynamic assessment and report writing but it should be subsequent to the same funding being invested in video interaction with parents and the educationalists that know the child best. Reports written following video work then reflect what has been discussed, implemented, observed and integrated into the child's context from the collaborative partnership with the team understanding how to focus on emerging skills and developing a learning self-identity.

Questioning received wisdom

The opportunity to work with the skills of so many individuals through video has enlightened my working practice and has led me to seriously question our role as speech and language therapists and the philosophy and concepts behind much of our professional practice. It appears to me that much of our work is isolationist in its focus on specific 'diagnosis', and misinformed in its perception that a specialism is related to that diagnosis rather than the specialism being working with others through interaction. We don't specify treatment approaches based on the sex or colour of the client, but we still arrange services based on what we perceive to be the presenting condition.

As Coupe O'Kane and Goldbart (1998) say, "Traditional therapy based on grammarian perspective and behaviour modification: modelling, shaping, imitation, prompting and fading, forward and backward chaining and training with the use of tangible reinforcers have their uses, but they limit the opportunity for real communication" (p.28). Therapy which is structured along the lines of stimuli, where the learner is required to produce a predetermined response, removes the child's essential unique contribution 'unknowability' (Zembylas, 2007, p.36) and consequent motivation for participation.

There continue to be many models of therapy in which the focus appears to be gleaning information rather than analysing strategies that support the child, where clients are categorised by their perceived needs (based on a short child–therapist assessment and medical categorisation), placed on waiting lists and provided with irregular 'therapy' or indirect therapy which due to its sparse nature, cannot have an effect on the child's patterning system. This feeds the anxiety of the adults in the child's environment and reinforces the concept that the child requires different management, potentially compounding the child's difficulty. For the majority of children, a short course of video therapy, placing parents at the heart of their success and providing both of them with self-confidence, would resolve any ongoing issues, empower the adult to discuss the child's strengths and needs with confidence and would ensure that for many they are not perceived as vulnerable or as having additional needs on entering school. For those children with longer-term communication difficulties, working through parents from the outset means they are an ongoing optimum resource, the collaboration of skills working both ways for the duration of speech and language therapy involvement.

I struggle with some of the received wisdoms of speech and language therapy practice, e.g., working with clients one to one with traditional therapy, focusing on linguistically- or phonologically-based materials, facilitating responses, modelling strategies to parents or carers and practitioners in adult/therapist-led activities, leaving 'programmes' of activities and strategies, and working in segregated services that espouse multidisciplinary working and holding numerous meetings amongst professionals but continuing to work with clients individually.

For ourselves as therapists

The concepts of attachment and attunement permeate every area of our role as therapists, peer professionals, supervisors and managers. The core of speech and language therapy is the relationship that the therapist fosters with the client. This is established almost immediately on meeting. McCluskey (2005) has been able to demonstrate that in using the same principles of 'empathic attunement' (identified earlier in relation to attachment theory), with the parents, i.e., through body language and non-verbal means, we are able to have an immediate therapeutic effect on a person we have just met, and that if we fail to attune with empathy "the situation becomes non-therapeutic and the client is left feeling misunderstood, unrecognized and often angry" (Heard et al., 2009, p.xvi). Interestingly, face watching and mirroring are fundamental to this process between adults, as is being mindful of the principles of interaction through eye contact, waiting, listening, repeating, reflecting back and scaffolding information that is timely, specific and commensurate with the adult's understanding and observation.

Fooke and Askeland (2007) note that "current workplace cultures work against critical reflection as they become more and more procedure and regulation based" (p.7). Unfortunately, procedure does not influence change. Having managed an early years speech and language therapy service, I strongly believe that the service is far more cost efficient if the team is highly skilled, confident and reflective. The only way to ensure this is to establish high levels of supervision within every team, where the supervision is based on attunement and 'reflective practice' (Schön, 1983). Video interaction therapy is highly skilled and can be tiring. It necessitates a high level of self-awareness in the therapist. Creating and holding a learning space requires a climate or culture of support that the learner can trust to hold them over time (Kolb and Kolb, 2005). Deep learning and understanding is facilitated by deliberate, recursive practice on areas that are related to the learner's goals (Keeton, Sheckley and Griggs, 2002) and should be part of any team's continuing professional development through video reflective supervision. Discussion is all well and good, but in supporting parents and professionals in reflecting on their interaction timing we as a profession need to be fully aware of our own. As Stengelhofen (1993) states, "the difficulty is to find out which parts are purely espoused (talked about) and which parts are actually used in solving the problems of practice" (p.12). This concept is universal regardless of the stage of learning we are at and the profession or role we are in. There is often a marked discrepancy in what we say and think we do and what we actually do. Video provides the bridge through conscious experience and allows us to become meta-cognitively aware (Flavell, 1979) of how we are thinking and addressing issues about what we do.

The more we know about ourselves through our own self-reflection, the more we can influence others. There needs to be a focus within the team on self-knowledge and self-reflection in which people are willing to express themselves within a systematised structure of support. By holding self-reflective video at the core (Cummins and Hulme, 1997) we can develop a staff culture that enjoys discussion about clients, regularly involves presentations and naturally develops knowledge, understanding, motivation and mentors, avoiding inertia and contributing to and relishing new developments. This in turn cultivates individuals' feelings of vitality and job satisfaction, which in turn is highly motivational for clients. Quality provision through highly-skilled professionals has a profound impact on the outcomes of children in therapy. It is easily possible to re-allocate funds to ensure high levels of supervision and support in order to support those involved in each child's daily lives in order to optimise funding and resources. If teams are unable to offer such levels of supervision themselves such support is on offer through Skype, action learning sets and social media.

I believe that our models of service delivery should focus on the following principles, whatever the client group:

- Behave in a way you would like to be treated.

- Ensure that the individual feels vital and the source of the interaction.

- Focus on interaction as a priority.

- Work through those who know the client best.

- Momentarily strip down the process and timing of the interaction.

- Be confident in the role of silence.

- Follow the signals of the client and moderate your own as a consequence.

- Support with visual props and environmental systematization.

- Trust the individual to self-resource and enjoy their creativity.

- Relish in the child, the parent and the educator's increasing independence and autonomy.

- Place self-reflection through video at the core of what you do.

Summary

Speech and language therapy is sharing experience, knowledge and understanding through a facilitating relationship based on attunement, respect, trust, empathy and humour with the client and their carers at the heart. It involves self-awareness, self-reflection and self-monitoring within the therapist, the client and the client's carers. It should be transformative.

It is a process whereby the client, the family and ourselves are enabled to understand what is happening to each individual and what they can do to support themselves and how they can educate the environment to support them. It provides an opportunity to optimise connections in the child, their parents, their environment and in other relationships.

In this current political climate, 'funds' are limited and competition for those funds from different professional groups fierce. This needs to be the case. Do we believe that what we are currently offering has an impact? Do we know which aspects of the service have most impact and, if not, what would we need to do to our service and within ourselves to ensure that it does? Are we genuinely comprehensive, cost efficient and measurable? We need to prove ourselves to be invaluable through being explicit in our knowledge. We need to specify what we have to offer in addition to other services and as distinct from other services and to be honest about policies and procedures that do not work and roles that can be fulfilled by someone else. We need to make sure that we are not using lack of funds as an excuse for poor practice or for diluting what we believe in. Dilution leads to inefficacy. If we cannot effect change with a client then we should not be involved. We must be mindful of the 'images' we convey, prioritising the process of supporting clients' independence through self-regulation, interaction, self-knowledge, learning self-identity, self-esteem, resilience and robustness so that they and their families can support themselves and really enjoy the benefits of interaction and communication. We must move away from a medical model and stop saying that we do not believe in it whilst carrying on propagating it.

As a profession, we need to analyse how we can be more effective and efficient for more clients, being ruthlessly reflective with ourselves, challenging our own concepts of therapy, outcomes, our own forms of service delivery, policies, procedures and administration. This needs to be done through clear systems of support, supervision and continuing professional development that offer the opportunity for deep learning rather than just surface understanding. We need to question, debate, theorise, and adapt, making the most of successful client-centred systems and letting go of ineffective practices. We need to make the most of knowledge from other disciplines and, most importantly, make the most of the skills of our clients and their families. Through the use of video we need to fully re-evaluate our roles and responsibilities and be clear about the unique, fascinating and highly rewarding role of the speech and language therapist.

References

Alt, M., Meyers, C. & Ancharski, A. (2012) Using principles of learning to inform language therapy and design for children with specific language impairment. *International Journal of Language and Communication Disorders*, 47(5), 487–498.

Ainsworth, M. & Bell, S.M. (1970) Attachment, exploration, and separation: Illustrated by the behavior of one-year-olds in a strange situation. *Child Development*, 41, 49–67.

Ainsworth, M., Blehar, M., Waters, E. & Wall, S. (1978) *Patterns of Attachment. A Psychological Study of the Strange Situation*. Hove: Psychology Press.

Banks, A. (2011) The mythic reality of the autonomous individual: Developing the capacity to connect. *Zygon*, 46(1).

Bateson, M.C. (1975) Mother-infant exchanges: The epigenesis of conversational interaction. In D. Aaronson & R.W. Rieber (Eds) *Developmental Psycholinguistics and Communication Disorders*. Annals of the New York Academy of Sciences, Vol. 263. New York: New York Academy of Sciences, pp.101–113.

Beebe, B., Knoblauch, S., Rustin, J. & Sorter, D. (2003) A comparison of Meltzoff, Trevarthen, and Stern. *Psychoanalytic Dialogues*, 13(6), 809–836.

Botterill, W. & Kelman, E. (2009) Palin parent-child interaction. In B. Guitar,& R. McCauley (Eds) *Treatment of Stuttering: Established and Emerging Interventions*. Baltimore: Lippincott Williams and Wilkins, pp.63–90.

Bowlby, J. (1969) *Attachment and Loss, Vol. 1: Attachment*. New York: Basic Books.

Brennan, S., Galati, A. & Kuhle, A. (2010) Two minds, one dialog: Coordinating speaking and understanding. In B. Ross (Ed.) *The Psychology of Learning and Motivation* 53, Burlington: Academic Press, pp.301–344.

Bretherton, I. & Munholland, K.A. (1999) Internal working models in attachment: A construct revisited. In J. Cassidy and P. Shaver (Eds), *Handbook of Attachment: Theory, Research and Clinical Application*. New York: Guilford Press, pp.89–111.

Brown, L.V. (2007). *Psychology of Motivation*. New York: Nova Science Publishers.

Caldwell, M., Rudolph, K., Troop-Gordon, W. & Kim, D. (2004) Reciprocal influences among relational self-views, social disengagement, and peer stress during early adolescence. *Child Development*, 75(4), 1140–1154.

Camarata, S.M., Nelson, K.E. & Camarata, M. (1994) Comparison of conversational-recasting and imitative procedures for training grammatical structures in children with specific language impairment. *Journal of Speech and Hearing Research*, 37, 1414–1423.

Clark, H.H. & Brennan, S.E. (1991) Grounding in communication. In L.B. Resnick, J.M. Levine & S.D. Teasley (Eds) *Perspectives on Socially Shared Cognition*. Washington, D.C.: American Psychological Association, pp.127–149.

Cooper, J., Moodley, M. & Reynell, J. (1978) *Helping Language Development: A Developmental Programme for Children with Early Language Handicaps*. London: Edward Arnold Publishers.

Coupe O'Kane, J. & Goldbart, J. (1998) *Communication Before Speech, Development and Assessment*. London: David Fulton Publishers Ltd.

Cummins, K. & Hulme, S. (1997) Video, a reflective tool. *Speech & Language Therapy in Practice Magazine*, 4–7.

Cummins, K. & Hulme,S. (2001) Managing preschool children in community clinics. In M. Kersner & J. Wright (Eds) *Speech and Language Therapy, the Decision Making Process when Working with Children*. London: David Fulton Publishers Ltd., pp.53–62.

Demos, E.V. (1989). Resiliency in infancy. In T.F. Dugan & R. Coles (Eds) *The Child in our Times: Studies in the Development of Resiliency*. New York: Brunner/Mazel, pp.3–22.

Doidge, N. (2007). *The Brain that Changes Itself: Stories of Personal Triumph from the Frontiers of Brain Science*. New York: Viking.

Dunst, C.J., Lowe, L.W. & Bartholomew, P.C. (1990). Contingent social responsiveness, family ecology, and infant communicative competence. *NSSLHA Journal*, 17, 39–49.

Durkin, K. & Conti-Ramsden, G. (2010) Young people with specific language impairment: A review of social and emotional functioning in adolescence. *Child Language Teaching and Therapy*, 26(2), 105–121.

Feldman, R. (2007) Parent–infant synchrony and the construction of shared timing; physiological precursors, developmental outcomes, and risk conditions. *Journal of Child Psychology and Psychiatry*, 48(3/4), 329–352.

Fishbane, M. (2007). Wired to connect: Neuroscience, relationships and therapy. *Family Process*, 46(3), 395–412.

Flavell, J.H. (1979) Metacognition and cognitive monitoring: A new area of cognitive-developmental inquiry. *American Psychologist*, 34, 906–911.

Florez, I.R. (2011) Developing young children's self-regulation through everyday experiences. *Young Children*, 66(4), 46–51.

Fonagy, P., Gergely, G.& Target M. (2007) The parent–infant dyad and the construction of the subjective self. *Journal of Child Psychology and Psychiatry*, 48(3/4), 288–328.

Fook ,J. & Askeland, G.U. (2007) Challenges of critical reflection: 'Nothing ventured, nothing gained'. *Social Work Education*, 26(5), 520–533.

Gallese, V., Keysers, C. & Rizzolatti, G. (2004) A unifying view of the basis of social cognition. *Trends in Cognitive Sciences*, 8, 396–403.

Gerhardt, S. (2004) *Why Love Matters: How Affection Shapes a Baby's Brain*. Hove: Brunner Routledge

Gutstein, S. (2009) *The RDI Book. Forging New Pathways for Autism, Asperger's and PDD with the Relationship Development Intervention Programme*. Connections Center Publishing.

Heard, D. & Lake, B. (1997) *The Challenge of Attachment for Caregiving*. London: Routledge.

Heard, D., Lake, B. & McCluskey, U. (2009) *Attachment Therapy with Adolescents and Adults: Theory and Practice Post Bowlby*. London: Karnac Books.

Holler, J. & Wilkin, K. (2011) Co-speech gesture mimicry in the process of collaborative referring during face-to-face dialogue. *Journal of Nonverbal Behaviour*, 35, 133–153.

Keeton, M.T., Sheckley, B. G. & Griggs, J.K. (2002) *Effectiveness and Efficiency in Higher Education*. Dubuque, IA: Kendall/Hunt.

Kelman, E. & Schneider, C. (1994) Parent-child interaction: An alternative approach to the management of children's language difficulties. *Child Language Teaching and Therapy*, 10(1), 81–96.

Kennedy, H., Landor, M. & Todd, L. (2011) *Video Interaction Guidance: A Relationship-based Intervention to Promote Attunement, Empathy and Wellbeing*. London: Jessica Kingsley Publishers.

Kolb, A.Y. & Kolb, D.A. (2005) The Kolb learning style inventory. Version 3.1: 2005 Technical Specifications. Haygroup: Experience Based Learning Systems Inc.

McCluskey, U. (2005) *To Be Met as a Person: The Dynamics of Attachment in Professional Encounters*. London: Karnac Books.

Miller, J. & Stiver, I. (1997) *The Healing Connection*. Boston: Beacon Press.

Molden, D.C. & Dweck, C.S. (2006) Finding "meaning" in psychology: A lay theories approach to self-regulation, social perception and social development. *American Psychologist*, 61(3), 192–203.

Mundy, P., Kasari, C., Sigman, M.,& Ruskin, E. (1995) Non-verbal communication and early language acquisition in children with Down syndrome and in normally developing children. *Journal of Speech and Hearing Research*, 38, 157–167.

Nind, M. & Hewett, D. (2005) *Access to Communication*, 2nd ed. London: David Fulton Publishers Ltd.

Prizant, B.M., Wetherby, A.M., Rubin, E., Laurent, A.C. & Rydell, P. (2006) *The SCERTS Model: A Comprehensive Educational Approach for Children with Autism Spectrum Disorders*. Baltimore, MD: Paul H. Brookes Publishing.

Ramachandran, V.S. (2011) *The Tell-Tale Brain: Unlocking the Mystery of Human Nature: Tales of the Unexpected from Inside your Mind*. London: Windmill Books.

Rice, M., Sell, M. & Hadley, P. (1991) Social interactions of speech and language impaired children. *Journal of Speech and Hearing Research*, 34, 1299–1307.

Roberts, M. & Kaiser, A. (2011) The effectiveness of parent-implemented language interventions: A meta-analysis. *American Journal of Speech-Language Pathology*, 20, 180–199.

Saxton (2005) "Recast" in a new light: Insights for practice from typical language studies. *Child Language Teaching and Therapy*, 21(1), 23–38.

Schön, D. (1983) *The Reflective Practitioner*. New York: Basic Books.

Schore, A.N. (2001) The effects of a secure attachment relationship on right brain development, affect regulation, and infant mental health. *Infant Mental Health Journal*, 22, 7–66.

Siegel, D.J. (2012) *The Developing Mind. How Relationships and the Brain Interact to Shape Who We Are,* 2nd ed. New York: Guilford Press.

Schore, A. (2003) *Affect Regulation and the Repair of the Self*. New York: Norton.

Stengelhofen, J. (1993) *Teaching Students in Clinical Settings*. London: Chapman and Hall.

Stern, D. (1985) *The Interpersonal World of the Infant: A View from Psychoanalysis and Developmental Psychology*. London: Karnac Books.

Stern, D. (2002) *The First Relationship, Infant and Mother*. Cambridge: Cambridge University Press.

Trevarthen, C. (1993) The self born in intersubjectivity: The psychology of an infant communicating. In U. Neisser (Ed.) *The Perceived Self: Ecological and Interpersonal Sources of Self-knowledge*. New York: Cambridge University Press, pp.121–173.

Trevarthen, C. & Aitken, J. (2001) Infant intersubjectivity: Research, theory, and clinical applications. *Journal of Child Psychology and Psychiatry*, 42(1), 3–48.

Vygotsky, L.S. (1962) *Thought and Language*. Cambridge, MA: MIT Press.

Vygotsky, L.S. (1978) *Mind and Society: The Development of Higher Mental Processes*. Cambridge, MA: Harvard University Press.

Wetherby, A., Alexander, D. & Prizant, B. (1996) The ontogeny and role of repair strategies. In A. Wetherby, S. Warren & J. Reichle (Eds) *Transitions in Prelinguistic Communication: Preintentional to Intentional and Presymbolic to Symbolic*. Baltimore: Paul H. Brookes, pp.135–159.

Wetherby, A., Prizant, B. & Hutchinson, T. (1998) Communicative, social/affective, and symbolic profiles of young children with autism and pervasive developmental disorders. *American Journal of Speech-Language Pathology*, 7(2), 79–91.

Wilson, E.O. (1998) *Consilience: The Unity of Knowledge*. New York: Knopf.

Yoder, P., Camarata, S. & Gardner, E. (2005) Treatment effects on speech intelligibility and length of utterance in children with specific language and intelligibility impairments. *Journal of Early Intervention*, 28, 34–49.

Zembylas, M. (2007) *Five Pedagogies, a Thousand Possibilities. Struggling for Hope and Transformation in Education*. Rotterdam: Sense Publishers.

5 A sociocultural perspective on speech and language therapy and education: Overlaps between the two professions

Deirdre Martin and Jane Stokes

This chapter discusses learning language, with a focus on learning, in contexts of working with children, adolescents and adults with speech, language and communication needs and difficulties. The discussion identifies important similarities and contrasts in ways of understanding language learning which are shaped and informed as much by theoretical understandings of language learning as by national and professional policies and professional practices. The chapter opens with a discussion of language learning from a sociocultural perspective, which is more frequently found in education rather than a cognitive perspective which is dominant in speech and language therapy. The second part discusses similarities and contrasts across understandings and practices of speech and language therapists and teachers, through the views of students on a postgraduate programme which includes teachers who re-train to become speech and language therapists.

Introduction

The quizzical problem with language disabilities is that *language* is both the tool for learning and the artefact that must be developed. It is clear how potentially devastating language learning difficulties can be for the intellectual, social and emotional development of children and adults with speech language and communication needs (SLCN).

The following discussion of language learning in speech and language therapy concerns the *process of learning*, where both parties, therapist and learner, change in the process of therapy/learning. The discussion sets out key concepts in sociocultural approaches to learning, and goes on to discuss three important ideas underpinning sociocultural accounts of language and learning, offered by Halliday (1979/1980): *learning language, learning about language,* and *learning through language.* These three knowledges of language highlight the relevance of the primary role of language in curriculum learning for speech and language therapists working with learners with speech and language disabilities. Halliday's ideas capture a more extended notion of language development that is beginning to emerge in speech and language therapy research and practice.

Mind and mediation

Speech and language therapy is still largely informed by medical and cognitive psychology, where learning is often perceived through a prism of biological development and maturation. The relationship between brain, mind and language is central to theories of language and learning. From a sociocultural perspective, mediation is the making of mind, that is, it concerns the relationship between the biological brain and the social, cultural and historical world. Mediation in speech and language therapy is the collaboration between therapist and child or adult with speech language and communication needs, to achieve new language learning. Intervention-learning is achieved in a time-space where the learner is capable of learning, that is, the zone of proximal development (zpd). Together, therapist and learner must gauge this space for new learning to be achieved, using the Dynamic Assessment method (e.g., Gutierrez-Clellen and Peña, 2001). Mediation in intervention with socially and culturally shared signs develops representational meanings in the learner's mind. In cases of the most severe language difficulties, developmental or as a result of brain damage, language and communication can be developed by alternative mediational tools such as sign language and augmentative communication systems.

Learning language

Language learning as development in very young children is often interpreted through maturation, where the biological genome drives language development, such that substantial physical, social or emotional disruption is necessary for language development to become delayed or disordered (Bishop and Mogford,

1993). An alternative interpretation is offered through sociocultural approaches where the encouragement of children's social engagement in learning of language is foregrounded.

> A sociocultural approach emphasises that language is socially constructed rather than internally intrinsic, language is both referential and constructive of social reality and notions of distributed and assisted activity in contrast to individual accomplishment.
>
> (Thorne, 2000, p.223)

Let us explore this quotation further to tease out the implications for speech and language therapy. Language learning is first social and then individual. An infant cries and flaps her arms and immediately gains her parent's attention (or a nearby Other) who picks her up, gives comfort and whatever else is required to soothe her. A sociocultural interpretation is that the adult has attributed meaning – an urgent request for help – to the infant's *ad hoc* noise and movements, and the child has learned that her *ad hoc* noises and physical movements gain a response to her need. Children usually soon learn to make their cries and body movements directed and intentional. What is important in this familiar scenario is that both parent/adult and child learn how to do the interaction. They transform an idiosyncratic event to a purposeful social interaction, so the interaction becomes conscious and intentional. The cry and arm movements become communicative signs between child and carer, and usually become more symbolic – a language – so that the vocalisation alone is used to communicate with other carers (Tomasello, Kruger and Ratner, 1993).

Furthermore, progressing from making a cry and arm flapping to *using* a cry and arm flapping to gain attention is transformational for the child's development. The child has transcended from *being an object* of communication to *becoming a subject*, a communicative agent in her world. This important transformation is part of the transcendence to being more socially and culturally human, which is the purpose of learning (Vygotsky, 1978, 1987), and speech and language therapy assessment and intervention.

Vygotsky placed communication and language learning in social, cultural and historical contexts. Culturally, the child has learned in this interaction that someone comes in response to her cry and arm waving. That is, she has become conscious of how the people around her know how to behave towards her and to each other, and she in turn learns how to respond to them. Children learn the ways "by which the 'instructions' about how humans should grow are carried from one generation to the next" (Bruner, 1986, p.135). Bruner uses the analogy that as the human genome transmits biological characteristics across generations, so social characteristics are passed on through 'culture' and cultural practices. Linguistic anthropologists Ochs and Schieffelin (1984) in their work in communities across countries, established that families and carers socialise their children to and through the use of language in very different ways to achieve social, emotional and linguistic learning within the cultural-historical frame of the family and social group.

An historical perspective is recognised in case history taking by speech and language therapists, concerning an interest and exploration of how children, or older people, have developed their communicative skills and practices. Case history taking can be a performance of checking biological and cognitive developmental milestones, and it can also be an observation and exploration of the family's communicative practices in one or more languages and literacies with and around the child, young person or adult. Also the association between communication and emotional development enhances the interpretation of interactions in young children and their parents, particularly mothers. By identifying these early forms of communication, such as the cry-response interactions, as an important feature, Trevarthen (1979) noted that absence of, or difficulties in, development of these kinds of social and emotional communications between mothers and children was an indicator for later difficulties in children's emotional development.

Although behaviourism has been discounted as an adequate explanation for developmental language learning, it continues to be used as an approach to teaching–learning communication skills with those with severe communication needs. Behaviourism posits that individual learning is achieved through repetitive practice of non-conscious behaviours and motivation is maintained by immediate and later extended reward systems. Studies with Picture Exchange Communication System (PECS, Frost and Bondy, 1985) suggest that students can learn to use these signs spontaneously for meaningful, situated communication (Bondy and Frost, 2001). While a sociocultural reading of language learning is profoundly different from behaviourist explanations of language development, there may be examples of the PECS tool being used which evidence Thorne's "notions of distributed and assisted activity" (Thorne, 2000).

From a strong cognition-maturational perspective, Piaget (e.g., 1962) and others argue that cognitive development precedes and enables language development. In contrast, a sociocultural perspective sees communication, language and other symbolic sign systems, such as literacy, *leading development*, where cognitions follow. It is through language in social interaction that shared, distributed, and individual cognitions develop. As children and older learners internalise language, they use language as a tool for thinking. Children with severe language difficulties use the haptic medium of signing, e.g., the Makaton Language Programme (Grove and Walker, 1990) or PECS, to 'say' the word, and finally use the word on its own and relationally with other words.

Revisiting Thorne's quotation, the sociocultural perspective places language learning, with words, signs and literacy, as occurring first *outside* the child or student, or older adult, and through modified interaction for mediation, the social language is drawn in and becomes internalised by the learner as both thought and the language system. This perspective is immensely important in speech and language therapy.

Referring to speech and language difficulties, a sociocultural approach to understanding language emphasises the interconnection between the social, cultural, historical and emotional in the development of the child and the important others in her/his communication world. When interconnections are not built up, or even fragment, then difficulties arise in speech, language and communication and possibly wider development. There are implications for speech and language therapists in case history gathering. While the biological aspects of development are important, a sociocultural orientation tracks the path of interactional development of child, mother and important others, across social, cultural, historical and emotional interactions in the language(s) of the home. Speech and language therapists and other professionals can develop these skills working with multilingual families. Linguistic anthropological studies show that interactions are most important in developing children's communication and language, rather than one particular, cultural and social method of child rearing (e.g., Ochs and Schieffelin, 1984).

Learning about language

The second of Halliday's language knowledges is metacognitive knowledge of language. That is, metalinguistic knowledge is being able to examine language as an entity in itself. Metalinguistic approaches seek to make language learning conscious to the learner, where language becomes a manageable tool that they can develop to understand others and to express their thoughts. Raising consciousness of both the problem and the solution is a scaffold for learners to develop learning strategies which support their learning, and to build linguistic and cognitive resources for their communication and wider learning. Developing metalinguistic knowledge in multilingual speakers/learners with language difficulties is important groundwork. Metalinguistic knowledge has become better understood through its use in pedagogy for phonological awareness in early literacy skills. Metalinguistic knowledge is an important tool in speech and language therapists' assessment of, and intervention for, learners' awareness of speech sounds in contexts of articulation and phonological delay and difficulties. The speech difficulties programmes Metaphon (Dean et al., 1995) and the Nuffield Centre Dyspraxia Programme (2014), are good examples of this approach. Beyond metacognition of speech, speech and language therapists develop metalinguistic knowledge of morphology, grammar, vocabulary, and pragmatics. Narratives are widely used as an assessment and intervention tool for raising awareness of language and language use. Therapy approaches also involve explicit teaching to raise awareness and meta-awareness of communicative intent for those with social language difficulties, such as Asperger's Syndrome and autism. It is a therapy approach in dysfluency, and in therapy with older people following brain damage. An important characteristic of metacognitive and metalinguistic therapy approaches is their capacity to empower young learners and adults with a consciousness not only of the difficulties they may have but also of the tools and strategies they can become equipped with to manage them.

Learning through language

The third knowledge of language that Halliday, and also Bernstein (1999), identified is the role of language in academic school learning. Bernstein's work, influenced by Vygotsky's ideas, identifies the importance of language as a tool for higher order thinking. He was concerned with how children learn to move from the 'common sense' talk of understanding their everyday lives (horizontal discourse) to the concepts of curriculum subject domains (vertical discourse). While Bernstein saw poverty/social class as an exclusionary force for children's learning through language, there are concerns currently in meeting the pedagogic challenges of inclusion policies in mainstream classrooms for children with special educational needs (SEN) and learners of English as an additional language (EAL).

Whilst speech and language therapy has focused mainly on provision for younger learners, it is becoming increasingly necessary that speech and language therapists' knowledge of learning through language is needed to support learners at secondary school and college level. This aspect of language learning is studied by speech and language therapists working in mainstream secondary contexts (e.g., Nippold 2007; Joffe and Black 2012). In the UK, there are professional boundaries separating speech and language therapists and the teaching profession that need to be further explored through studies of inter-professional learning.

Collaborative learning

This section presents inter-professional collaboration as learning: *learning to work together* and *working to learn together*. Most speech and language therapists work with a range of professionals in education and health contexts to meet clients'/patients' needs as well as working with learners with communication needs from both monolingual and culturally and linguistically diverse families. A focus on learning highlights that practitioners are continuing to develop expertise in this area.

What are the problems? Collaboration among professionals can result in services which overlap, or underlap, or become fragmented in addressing the speech language and communication needs of children, adolescents and adults. This section examines three models of inter-professional work that are prevalent in education and health provisions through a lens of sociocultural activity theory of organisational learning, from a post-Vygotskian perspective.

Learning to collaborate

Here are illustrations of three types of 'learning to collaborate' with different emphases on following professional scripts, roles and procedures to meet learners' needs in collaborative intervention.

Coordination

Scenario 1 Multilingual learners with language and learning needs have three sessions a week: one from the speech and language therapist who supports their phonological difficulties, another from the literacy specialist to support reading, and a third from the EAL teacher to support development of vocabulary for curriculum learning. In this model of collaboration, each professional meets the learners' needs while maintaining their own discrete professional script, their role and intervention approach. They may correspond termly to coordinate their work around the learners.

Cooperation

Scenario 2 Multilingual learners with language and learning needs have three sessions a week where the speech and language therapist works on the phonology of key curriculum vocabulary, the literacy specialist supports reading, spelling and writing of key curriculum vocabulary, and the EAL teacher supports conceptual meaning of key curriculum vocabulary. They meet termly to plan the key curriculum language and vocabulary for the learners. In this model of collaboration, the three 'actors' are led by the needs of the learner to develop a shared 'object' of their practice, yet they maintain the hidden script of their professional roles.

Communication

Scenario 3 Multilingual learners with language and learning needs have learning support three sessions a week on a fortnightly rota from each professional: speech and language therapist, literacy specialist and EAL teacher. The speech and language therapist, EAL teacher and literacy specialist meet during the term to plan in some detail for the learners' phonological, reading and curriculum language needs. They agree learning aims, objectives, and methods of teaching-learning that they will draw on in the sessions, and agree a method of recording each learner's engagement and achievements. The fortnightly teaching rota aims to achieve more consistency across specialist pedagogies with the learners.

Arrangements for inter-professional collaboration are mediated by national and local policies, and professional cultures. Yet, bearing in mind Thorne's "notions of distributed and assisted activity in contrast to individual accomplishment" (2000), these examples illustrate possibilities for collective learning to best meet learners' needs, within resourcing constraints.

This half of the chapter has taken a sociocultural lens to focus key aspects of speech and language therapy practice, such as case history taking, understanding language learning in development, assessment, working in monolingual and multilingual settings, and working collaboratively with other professionals. Through this lens, learning can be understood as a primarily social activity which becomes individual, where language is *the* tool for learning. Speech and language therapists are often well positioned to be effective leaders and coordinators of inter-professional collaborative learning for a number of reasons, and probably most significantly because they are conscious of the importance of language and communication as tools for learning.

Overlaps between speech and language therapy and education

The need for speech and language therapists to understand more about the process of learning is a theme that has arisen in discussion with speech and language therapy students who come from the world of education. Traditionally, speech and language therapy curricula pay limited attention to learning theory, and less to the sociocultural aspects outlined above. Speech and language therapists in the UK are not educated alongside teachers, although they may both attend the same institutions. A significant number of postgraduate speech and language therapy students have experience working in education. On the programme run by the Universities at Medway, several have been class teachers, some have been special needs coordinators, and some have been head teachers, who have decided that they would like to specialise in the area of communication difficulties. This section of the chapter discusses their experience in making the change from teacher to speech and language therapist and reflects on the differences and similarities between the two professions. It draws on interviews carried out with seven such students after they had completed the programme and been working as speech and language therapists for a couple of years. In this section, we record the insights that they brought to the discussion. In bringing these to the fore, we gain more understanding of just exactly what is speech and language therapy and examine what we perhaps need to teach and focus on in pre- and post-registration education. We offer these reflections as observations that will be interesting to people who have taken this route into the profession or who are considering becoming speech and language therapists. We see these observations as contributions to the many- sided prism through which to look at the profession. It is recognised that some of the comments made are coloured by the fact that they come from people who have left teaching and therefore may have a slightly more negative view of it than those who stay in the profession. There is no attempt to counter the balance – the comments are presented as they were made, as stimuli for reflection. The conversations explored themes surrounding the overlap between education and speech and language therapy.

Are teaching and therapy the same thing? What are the common features and the key differences?

Those interviewed identified a number of similarities between the processes in therapy and the processes in teaching. Many of the principles underlying the two professions are shared.

Interviewees felt that teachers and speech and language therapists both look at baseline achievements and both measure progress in incremental steps. Both use the processes of scaffolding learning on prior learning. Both identify learning objectives and activities to work towards to achieve these.

Essential skills such as facilitation and feedback are shared across both professions, but those interviewed pointed to a significant difference. With speech and language therapy, a session is conceived more as a collaboration between therapist and child. The focus is on negotiating the content together, with shared aims made explicit. This is more challenging to do in a classroom context and does not fit so easily into the teacher–pupil relationship. This collaborative approach tends to be more embedded in the therapist–client relationship.

The skill of breaking down concepts into smaller steps is central to both professions, but the interviewees felt that the speech and language therapist had more developed skills in this area, especially in regard to language. When, for example, introducing new vocabulary in a classroom, the teacher starts from the standpoint that most children are able to absorb new vocabulary without much support so does not always know how to make this process easier for those who find it difficult. The teacher would present the word usually just once or twice, whereas the speech and language therapist would devote more time to supporting the child to understand it, giving them props, prompts and checking and rechecking understanding in a process of micro-scaffolding of the learning of language. There is not the time to do this as part of usual classroom activity. Speech and language therapists who had been teachers observed that it felt like a luxury to have the time to really listen to a child, unpick what was going on when they are finding language difficult and think through the best way to support that child. The onus on the teacher is to do the best for the whole class and this can mean that targets are less individualised.

The analysis and diagnostic skills that a speech and language therapist is expected to use are not part of a teacher's repertory. Interviewees reported that when they were teachers, there was simply not the time to spend on detailed analysis of communication, and this is an area where real collaboration is so valuable. Teachers are more used to looking at trends and cohorts across larger groups of children, whereas speech and language therapists are more used to looking at individuals. Teachers are not expected to know about stages of attention, stages of language development, how vocabulary develops or how phonological development interacts with phonics, for example. The interviewees felt that it is important for speech and language therapists to realise this and to be generous with their knowledge of these areas supporting the teachers in using the combined skills of therapists and teachers to work with children. The emphasis placed by teachers on literacy complements the focus on oral skills by therapists and, by joint working, ideas can be pooled. Several student practitioners who came from the world of education felt that speech and language therapists needed to understand more about how children learn to read, an area that is given little time in speech and language therapy curricula. Those who were teachers benefited from being able to combine these areas of knowledge and skills. They felt that speech and language therapists can support teachers to look at their own communication styles, which is rarely a focus in training teachers. The use of video, common practice in therapy, is not so widespread in training teachers. There was a feeling amongst the interviewees that it would be very beneficial for student teachers and student speech and language therapists to be taught alongside each other.

What are the differences in professional culture between teaching and speech and language therapy?

Those speech and language therapists who had been teachers commented that within speech and language therapy they felt that the client is more in control. Within teaching, the control of the teacher is given more importance and there are fewer options on the part of the child or young person in refusing to participate in the education process. Within speech and language therapy the client can refuse therapy. The client is more engaged in the setting of targets, whereas in education the targets are pre-set. Therapy can therefore be more client-centred and the direction of therapy can be individually tailored more closely than education can be. For this reason, the speech and language therapist needs to have a better ability to engage with the client, to collaborate in goal setting, and to minutely observe the response to therapy to ensure that it is effective.

Speech and language therapists who had been teachers reported that, as teachers, they felt that they were part of the apparatus within the school set up to meet the targets established by the school. There was a feeling among those who had been teachers that government drivers and expectations set the direction for teaching in a way that did not happen in speech and language therapy. Whereas therapy can start from where the child is, teaching must work towards targets pre-set by government policy. There is scope for tailoring these targets for the individual child but, ultimately, the individual targets are subordinate to overall curriculum objectives. Priorities are established by the inspection regime and by the senior management team. These externally driven targets do not exist for speech and language therapy. The work does not in the same way need to correspond to the school plan and business objectives. The interviewees felt that in schools there was more of a tendency in discussion about the pupils to dehumanise them, something that did not happen in speech and language therapy where the client-centred approach predominated. In teaching, the interviewees commented on the huge amounts of planning, record keeping and marking which depleted the energy of the teachers. The capacity to be spontaneous or to improvise was severely limited. By contrast, speech and language therapists are largely autonomous and independent of restrictions in how they achieve the mutually agreed aims for therapy. Therapists have more freedom to differentiate their work. Some ex-teachers felt that the political demands on teachers meant that the care and compassion was sometimes given less importance in education than in speech and language therapy.

The culture of supervision and support was one of the key differences between teaching and speech and language therapy. After the first year of teaching, the ex-teachers reported that in their experience there was limited opportunity for supervision or guidance. Although as teachers they were observed, the emphasis was more on looking for weaknesses in teaching rather than drawing on the positives. Reflective practice was also given much greater emphasis in speech and language therapy (see Chapter 1 of this book for further discussion of reflection).

Speech and language therapists' work is actively influenced by research and new approaches are subject to scrutiny as to the evidence base that underlies them. Those who were ex-teachers reported that they were less aware of research trends in education. They also felt that, whereas speech and language therapists were schooled in the importance of evidence-based practice, there was less of a focus on this in teaching. They contrasted the evidence base for teaching with that for speech and language therapists with one interviewee characterising the evidence base for teaching as being "data rich but information poor", i.e., that much data was collected but often not accessible to teachers in practice to support their professional development. In therapy, there was more of a focus on an individual, holistic approach for clients which did not play such an important part in teaching.

In becoming a speech and language therapist, what did you feel you had to give up in your identity as a teacher and what did you feel you did differently?

People who made the transition from teacher to therapist felt that they needed to adjust their working style and specifically reduce the directiveness of their approach. They had to work on moving from being directive to being responsive. They had to learn to follow the child's lead more. One ex-teacher commented that she had to learn to stay quiet, and felt that teachers had a tendency to intervene a lot earlier than a therapist if a child is finding something difficult. She felt that a teacher tended to want a child to succeed, and put steps in place to allow them to. A therapist, by contrast, waited to see how a child tackled a problem and by observing how the child managed difficulties, adapted their input accordingly. The therapist could be more flexible in the pacing of activities, the length of time they could spend on one target, whereas in teaching there were a predetermined number of targets to be met, goals to be attained. As ex-teachers, they had to learn to make the interaction more two-way, more of a dialogue than one directed by the teacher. This meant that they had to learn to say less, to ask less and to be less demanding generally of the child's responses. This was at times challenging for them. Having made the change from teacher to speech and language therapist, one interviewee reported that there was more time to observe children in more detail, to monitor their response to intervention. Therapists were able to spend longer gathering information and were able to broaden the scope of information gathered which as teachers they perhaps had not deemed relevant. There was a recognition that working in Early Years had more similarities with being a speech and language therapist.

In making the transition from teacher to therapist working with adults, one ex-teacher commented that in speech and language therapy there was more recognition that the client was the expert about their own condition. This perspective is absent in teaching, where it is the teacher who is the expert. This alters the power balance between client and therapist.

People who had been teachers were used to being able to assert authority and manage groups. These were important skills within teaching but not always useful in therapy where the emphasis tends to be more on seeing the student or pupil as an individual, and looking at their needs holistically. However, having been a teacher gave the speech and language therapists more confidence in managing behaviour, which is an area in which speech and language therapy students often feel inexperienced. Having been a teacher had given them confidence in being able to work with children and young people and to form relationships of trust with them. They were used to having to explain things using very clear communication and this aided their development as speech and language therapists.

People who had been teachers were also conscious that they were not using their performance skills as they had previously as class teachers. The satisfaction of being able to hold the attention of a class of children was no longer part of the role. There were fewer opportunities to get involved in celebrating festivals, joining in the cultural aspects of school life. There was a comfortable set of routines as a teacher whereas the daily life of a speech and language therapist is far less predictable, which brings its own pressures.

The stresses within speech and language therapy were reported to be different. Whereas in teaching, outcomes are measured continuously, in speech and language therapy, a system of consistent measurement of outcomes is still being developed. Several interviewees felt that this weakens the ability of the profession to demonstrate its impact. They commented that the measures can seem to be more subjective, so it can be harder for the speech and language therapist to prove his or her worth. Service pressures can result in services being cut, whereas teaching will not be cut in the same way. There was also a feeling that the role of the speech and language therapist is poorly understood, and therefore not always valued, whereas everyone understands the role of the teacher, or thinks they do. The profession of teacher was thought to be of higher status so that in becoming a speech and language therapist some of this status was sacrificed.

The interviewees felt that the teacher always has to consider the impact of a child's behaviour on the rest of the class – this is less of a concern to the speech and language therapist as the responsibility for behaviour management is not part of their role. The teacher is always considering the class dynamics as a whole, whereas this is of less concern to the speech and language therapist who may provide therapy with not enough consideration of this.

In becoming a speech and language therapist, the ex-teachers commented that they had had to develop their listening skills, which in education were accorded less importance than in speech and language therapy. Because of time constraints and class sizes, as a teacher there was less focus on the individual's contributions and there was less scope for really listening to these. The focus was on the performance of the individual pupils and how these contributed to the drivers of attainment.

In becoming a speech and language therapist, those who had been teachers were able to draw on their experience in a number of very positive ways. Obviously their knowledge of the education system gave them an advantage over others who had not had experience of the National Curriculum and special educational needs, policies and procedures. The experience of working in the statutory sector in a context that was highly politicised prepared them well for working in the health service. For ex-teachers, many of the essential skills were well developed – the creation of rapport, the support for learning, the setting of objectives, the reflective practice. The familiarity with stages of development and learning again put them at an advantage. These skills and knowledge were increased if the student was also a parent.

What do speech and language therapists need to know about teaching and teachers need to know about speech and language therapy?

The ex-teachers felt that speech and language therapists should understand aspects of the life of the teacher in order to make them better therapists. There was a feeling that the speech and language therapist should understand the time constraints that the teacher is under, the amounts of paperwork that formed part of their job. They needed to understand the pressure of the inspection regimes, OFSTED and the necessity for the teacher to perform and meet targets in a way that is not part of the speech and language therapy culture. Speech and language therapists need to understand that any work that they expect teachers to collaborate with must be realistic, and strategies that they suggest must be achievable in the classroom context. These ex-teachers were familiar with speech and language therapists coming in to their classrooms and recommending programmes of work that were neither relevant nor achievable. There was a realisation that programmes worked best when carried out by more experienced teachers and when resources to implement them were supplied.

Once students had completed the programme they felt that they could also advise teachers as to what they could learn about speech and language therapy. They felt it was important for teachers to understand that speech and language therapists put the learner at the centre of their work and that therapists were professional experts in their own field who were able to address complex and specific communication disorders.

Those who had been teachers felt that they were better speech and language therapists because of their teaching experience. Those who had returned to teaching felt that they were better teachers for having trained as speech and language therapists. They welcomed the fact that in training to become a speech and language therapist they had become more aware of their own communication style, better at identifying difficulties in children, and able to be more analytical and diagnostic in their approach. They became more aware of the difference in interaction styles, e.g., between asking questions and reflecting and better able to adapt their behaviour for each individual child.

They commented that teachers had a better sense of a community of practice with enormous amounts of shared experience on line, support in lesson plans and writing of targets. Teachers had more opportunities for continuous professional development than speech and language therapists. They felt that this was an area that could be better developed in speech and language therapy.

Conclusions

The transition between being a teacher and being a speech and language therapist is at times a natural one, with many overlapping skills and qualities. This brief series of interviews has highlighted some of the key similarities and differences and we hope will stimulate further discussion on the area, with more consideration given to the design of curricula and the potential for joint training of speech and language therapists and teaching at the pre-registration stage.

As a whole, this chapter has explored the importance of understanding more about the process of learning, specifically the sociocultural nature of learning. We have looked at how this relates to language learning and the difficulties some people experience. Through enhancing our understanding of learning, as speech and language therapists we can improve our collaboration with teachers, understand their perspectives and work towards common objectives more easily. The focus on the overlaps between teaching and speech and language therapy can help us to become more aware of the significance of the sociocultural contexts in which we both work, some of them shared and some of them individual to our respective professions.

References

Bernstein, B. (1999) Vertical and horizontal discourse: An essay. *British Journal of Sociology of Education*, 20(2), 157–173.

Bishop, D. & Mogford, K. (Eds) (1993) *Language Development in Exceptional Circumstances*. Hove: Lawrence Erlbaum.

Bondy, A.S. & Frost, L. (2001) The Picture Exchange Communication System. *Behaviour Modification*, 25(5), 725–744.

Bruner, J. (1986) *Actual Minds, Possible Worlds*. London: Harvard University Press.

Dean, E.C., Howell, J., Waters, D. and Reid, J. (1995) Metaphon: A metalinguistic approach to the treatment of phonological disorder in children. *Clinical Linguistics & Phonetics*, 9(1), 1–19.

Frost, L. & Bondy, A.S. (1985) *The Picture Exchange Communication System*. Newark, NJ: Pyramid Educational Consultants, Inc.

Grove, N. & Walker, M. (1990) The Makaton Vocabulary: Using manual signs and graphic symbols to develop interpersonal communication. *Augmentative and Alternative Communication*, 6(1), 15–28.

Gutierrez-Clellen, V.F. & Peña, E. (2001) Dynamic assessment of diverse children: A tutorial. *Language, Speech & Hearing Services in Schools*, 32(4), 212–224.

Halliday, M. (1979/1980) Three aspects of children's language development: Learning language, learning through language, learning about language. In Y. Goodman, M. Hausser & D. Strickland (Eds) *Oral and Written Language Development: Impact on Schools*, pp.7–19. Proceedings from the 1979 and 1980 IMPACT Conferences. Urbana, IL: International Reading Association and National Council of Teachers of English.

Joffe, V. & Black, E. (2012) The relationship between language, educational attainment and social, emotional and behavioural functioning in secondary school students with language and communication difficulties, *Language, Speech and Hearing Services in Schools*, 43, 461–473.

Nippold, M. (2007) *Later Language Development*, 3rd ed. Austin, TX: Pro-Ed.

Nuffield Centre Dyspraxia Programme NDP3® (2014) Eton: Nuffield Centre Dyspraxia Programme Ltd.

Ochs, E. & Schieffelin, B. (1984) Language acquisition and socialization: Three developmental stories and their implications. In R. Shweder & R.A. LeVine (Eds) *Culture Theory: Essays on Mind, Self, and Emotion*, pp.276–320. New York: Cambridge University Press.

Piaget, J. (1962) *The Language and Thought of the Child*. London: Routledge & Kegan Paul.

Thorne, S. (2000) Second language acquisition theory and the truth(s) about relativity. In J. Lantolf (Ed.) *Sociocultural Theory and Second Language Learning*, pp.219–243. Oxford: Oxford University Press.

Tomasello, M., Kruger, A. & Ratner, H. (1993) Cultural Learning. *Behavioural Sciences*, 16, 495–552.

Trevarthen, C. (1979) Communication and cooperation in early infancy: A description of primary intersubjectivity. In M. Bullowa (Ed.) *Before Speech: The Beginning of Interpersonal communication*, pp.321–347. Cambridge: Cambridge University Press,

Vygotsky, L.S. (1978*) Mind in Society: The Development of Higher Psychological Processes*. Cambridge, MA: Harvard University Press.

Vygotsky, L.S. (1987) *The Collected Works of L.S.Vygotsky. Vol 1: Problems of General Psychology*, including the volume *Thinking and Speech*. R.W. Rieber and A.S. Carton (Eds) (trans. N. Minick), pp.39–285. New York: Plenum Press.

6 Spirituality and speech and language therapy

Sophie MacKenzie

> "Healing of the psychosocial-biological is of itself insufficient to repair the existential disarray of the patient's life without recognition of the spiritual origins of that disarray."
> (Pellegrino, 2012)

Ask one hundred people to define the spirit or spirituality and you are likely to receive one hundred different definitions. Yet most people, I think, would not dispute the fact that there is a certain something, the essence of a being, which exists; whether we call it spirit, soul, connectedness or whatever, we are more than just body and mind.

In the Judeo-Christian tradition, we are told that before all else existed the spirit of God was 'hovering over the earth', a potential something from which all things derived. In the Old Testament, the spirit is referred to as 'ruach' or 'breath', and throughout the Bible the spirit is depicted as wind or fire, forces that are powerful, sustaining and pervasive.

The English word 'spirit' comes from the Latin 'spiritus', meaning 'breathing', so there is something about life force and essentiality about the term. I am reminded of a patient I worked with many years ago as a speech and language therapist. David, a man in his early 40s, had suffered a brainstem stroke which had left him completely paralysed, save for the ability to blink his left eye. His cognitive abilities, including his language skills, were intact, leaving him in the aptly named 'locked-in syndrome'. He was able to communicate very effectively by blinking his left eye – once for yes, twice for no. He was able to express more when an alphabet chart with listener scanning was introduced, and he was able to spell out novel thoughts and ideas. A film crew arrived at the hospital and I remember the question being put to David by one of the reporters, the question none of us healthcare professionals had dared to ask: "David, despite everything, do you still want to live?" He had lost so much – physical skills, autonomy, sexuality, role of father and husband, dignity. Despite all this loss, he blinked once. This, I believe, was the epitome of the human spirit, wanting connection with life despite devastating loss and suffering.

At points of despair or disruption in our lives, those nadir times when we experience acute loss of ability, health or personhood, we perhaps demonstrate our essential spirit but also need at these times to question, rail or doubt. Yet it is this very ability to express novel thoughts freely and comprehensively which is often denied the users of speech and language therapy services.

Imagine you have survived a catastrophic health event, an event which almost deprived you of your life. You survived but that event took away your former life, took away your previous life roles, took away some of your physical abilities – and took away your speech. How might you address the pressing existential questions post-trauma: why did I survive? What have I done to deserve this? What is the meaning of it all? And what might the consequences be of not being able to address these issues verbally?

Or suppose your child – your perfect child – is diagnosed with a communication impairment which means they will never be able to express themselves as freely as you or I. How might they communicate their angst at not being 'like the others' or their distress at finding life so hard? You, as the devastated parent, are able to seek solace from counsellors, healthcare professionals, peer support groups or priests. The child, on the other hand, may not have that verbal outlet.

Is it our role as speech and language therapists to attempt to understand the spiritual pain that our clients may undergo? Is it our role to facilitate their ability to express spiritual needs and distress? Or is it merely up to us to refer clients on to professional spiritual advisers such as chaplains, when we recognise spiritual distress?

Definitions of spirituality

Defining the term 'spirituality' can feel like trying to hold on to jelly; one minute you think you have a firm grasp of it, the next it has slipped through your fingers. But it is perhaps the nebulous quality to the term that gives it its strength and its usefulness. To some, it may refer to an organised religion to which they belong, complete with established liturgy, rules and sacred texts. For others, it might be a connection to other people or to nature, or a sense of transcendence or connection to an undefined 'other'.

I asked some speech and language therapy student practitioners what they understood by the term. "It's about knowing there's something greater than us," said one, and another, "It's about explaining the unexplainable."

Within health, numerous definitions abound, but most encompass the idea of hope, meaning and purpose in life, love and transcendence.

McSherry and Cash (2004, p.154) offer a taxonomy of spirituality (theistic, religious, language, ideologies, phenomenological, existential, quality-of-life and mystical), acknowledging that "the selection of definitions presented suggests that spirituality can be defined and interpreted differently because many of the definitions have several layers of meaning or defining characteristics." They offer a helpful suggestion that present-day spirituality falls into two distinct categories: that of the old, theocentric understanding of spirituality and that of the post-modern concepts of meaning, life purpose, creativity and relationships. Similarly, Bash (2004) talks of three categories of spirituality: non-theistic, theistic and what he terms the *via media*, that is a position halfway between having (a) God at the centre and not.

Origins of speech and language therapy as a profession

Speech and language therapy as a profession has its roots in the elocution movement of the 19th century (Duchan, 2001). Towards the end of the 1800s, a medical doctor who himself stuttered wrote one of the first US books on the subject of speech therapy (Potter, 1882); the emphasis in the early days seemed to have been very much on impairment and remediation. With the onset of the Second World War, there were sadly many examples of aphasia in soldiers sustaining penetrative head injuries. So it would appear that, as a profession, our roots were in fixing the bodily impairment, remediating the defect, sorting out the physical problem. Issues relating to the mind, or psychosocial factors, began to be addressed much later (e.g., Cruice et al., 2003). Spirituality as a concept in the therapies is only just beginning to gain prominence (Johnston and Mayers, 2005).

Nursing, by contrast, developed from a religious route. Hospitals began as charitable, religious institutions. Until relatively recently, nurses wore headdresses reminiscent of a nun's wimple and, even today, senior female nurses are referred to as 'sister'. Perhaps it is this link with religious charity which has made the nursing profession the forerunners amongst healthcare workers willing, able and confident to provide spiritual help to their patients (McSherry and Ross, 2010). Nurses have embraced the concept of the spiritual and routinely consider the spiritual needs, distress and wellbeing of their patients. The literature surrounding the spiritual within nursing has steadily grown throughout the last 20 years, with many books (McSherry and Ross, 2010), journal articles (McSherry, Cash and Ross, 2004) and journals (e.g., *Journal of Religion, Disability and Health*) being devoted to the subject. Nursing clerking forms have a section related to spirituality, which trained staff are expected to complete with patients on admission to hospital. Some nurses view discussing spirituality with their patients as an intrinsic and vital part of their role (Baldacchino, 2008). Others see their role as one of referrer on to another professional whose sole remit is spiritual, such as the hospital chaplain.

Person-centred care

Within healthcare in recent years, there has been a steady drive away from the reductionist view of patients being seen purely as a body. In speech and language therapy, as in all modern healthcare professions, emphasis is placed on an holistic approach to therapy and intervention, seeing the client as a whole person, in a person-centred way (Koubel and Bungay, 2008). Holism derives from the Greek word 'holos', meaning whole, so if we claim to be treating the

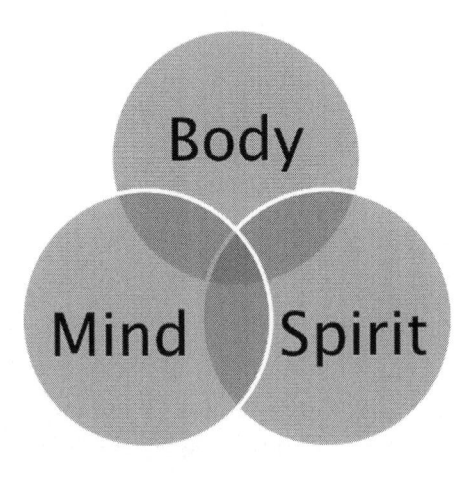

```
        ⎯ Spirit
   ⬤    ⎯ Mind
        ⎯ Body
```

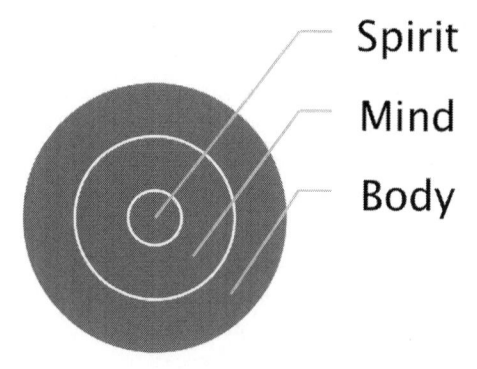

whole person in therapy (or in any caring profession), we need to consider all facets of our clients.

Therapy clients can be regarded as 'tripartite' in nature; that is, the essence of the individual comprises body, mind and spirit:

Frankl (2011) extends the concept of a person's wholeness being dependent on the interaction of all three aspects (body, mind, spirit), by suggesting that, not only should all aspects be present, but that the spiritual aspect creates the inner core around which the body and mind develop.

If we consider the client to be tripartite in nature, we can identify how speech and language therapists have become accustomed to assessing and intervening with the 'body' aspect. We have seen how, in the early years of the profession, the emphasis was on curing the lisp or stutter, providing exercises to improve the output of soldiers with aphasia. Impairment-based assessments and interventions still abound today, exemplified perhaps in the cognitive neuropsychological model of language processing and the assessments that partner it, such as the Psycholinguistic Assessment of Language Processing in Aphasia (Kay, Lesser and Coltheart, 1992) and the Comprehensive Aphasia Test (Swinburn, Porter and Howard, 2004). Using this model, the area of a client's language breakdown is accurately assessed and therapy provided to target that level of impairment. Similarly, in therapy for adults with acquired dysarthria, non-speech oromotor exercises are routinely implemented by speech and language therapists in an effort to improve rate, range and strength of movement of the articulators (Mackenzie, Muir and Allen, 2010). Speech and language therapists hoping to maximise the period of spontaneous recovery, providing the best support and environment in which spontaneous recovery and perhaps neuroplasticity (Vargha-Khadem et al., 1997) can take place, will advocate this emphasis on working with the body element of their tripartite clients.

In more recent years, although therapies with their focus on the body and impairment still maintain a large presence both in the efficacy literature and also in practice, emphasis has shifted slightly to incorporate the 'mind' within therapy. This is exemplified in the literature of the last 10 years, which has focused on, for example, the psychosocial elements of living with aphasia (Hilari et al., 2003). Issues of quality-of-life (Cruice et al., 2003) and identity (Ellis-Hill and Horn, 2000) have also rightly begun to be more thoroughly explored. Schemes such as the Conversation Partner Scheme, devised by the communication charity Connect UK, have sprung up over the last few years, in an attempt to address the need for people with communication impairment to live successfully with their disability.

But what of the 'spiritual' aspect of the tripartite client with a speech, language or communication problem? Do speech and language therapists address this aspect as part of their management of the tripartite client – and should they? If we consider Maslow's (1954) Hierarchy of Need, are we as speech and language therapists focusing only on those needs at the base of the pyramid (i.e., physiological and safety needs) and not being cognisant of our clients' need to progress to self-actualisation? Greenstreet (2006, p.13) believes that self-actualisation is linked to spirituality and is evidenced in "personal autonomy, self-acceptance, *open communication and interaction*" (my italics); perhaps the facilitative role of the speech and language therapist could play a part here.

Co-presence

The speech and language therapist could be viewed as a facilitative presence, accompanying the client on the rehabilitation journey towards communicative competence. Kvale and Brinkmann (2009) sketch the analogy of the traveller who accompanies an individual along a path. The traveller listens closely to the individual's story as they travel together, gently asking questions and passing comment, the better to understand the personal narrative. This is contrasted with the miner model, where the interviewer digs and probes to unearth information, in a systematic, investigative manner.

Vignette: L. E. Usher

L. E. Usher, a published author and poet who has been living with aphasia since 2008, generously shared with me some of her thoughts about spirituality in relation to her stroke story in interviews and in email correspondence.

Lindy's comprehension of spoken and written language is excellent but her expressive language has been affected by the stroke; she is able to produce single words and short phrases but presents with significant word-finding difficulties.

She is highly communicative, employing a variety of verbal and non-verbal communication strategies, including speech, writing, gesture and intonation.

Lindy talks and writes eloquently of her spiritual experiences, seemingly with no self-consciousness.

A notable theme is that of benevolent visions. Whilst in a post-stroke coma which lasted three days, Lindy describes how she is given a sense of peace by what she describes as angelic beings:

" Angels? [questioning intonation] I don't know…um…um…God? [questioning intonation] I don't know"

In a subsequent email, she seems more certain of the identity of these beings:

"I experience profound JOY. Angels: intense compassion and androgynous. The most real thing I have ever felt"

She contrasts the peace of the angels with the desperation she feels on waking from the coma, when she realises she has lost her communicative ability:

"me crying, crying [despairing intonation]"

During the coma, Lindy also saw her mother and her father, both of whom had died some years before. She describes these appearances of her parents as a 'barrier', preventing the work of Azreal, the Angel of Death with his sickle, who according to the Qur'an, takes the soul of the dying person and returns it to God.

Lindy talks about the miracle of surviving this catastrophic stroke, seemingly against all odds:

"I am Lazarus"

and she explores the idea of near-death experience and the effect on the brain.

Spirituality is evidently an important part of Lindy's life. She explains how she feels connected to God through nature:

"yeah…um…me walking…um…trees…um…grass…God"

Restitution, chaos, quest and the therapeutic journey

In his book *The Wounded Storyteller* (Frank, 1995), Arthur Frank, a medical doctor exploring both his own and others' illness narratives, identifies three distinct types of storytelling, namely restitution, chaos and quest. He describes how these different narrative types are told by patients "alternately and repeatedly". Interestingly, Frank equates the telling of the illness narrative as self-actualisation of sorts:

> Stories have to *repair* the damage that illness has done to the ill person's sense of where she is in life, and where she may be going. Stories are a way of redrawing maps and finding new destinations
>
> (Frank, 1995, p.53)

Storytelling is a powerful means of expression which can be denied our clients with communication difficulties.

Although Frank's narrative typology pertains to acute illness, I think it can also usefully be employed when considering disability, be that disability resulting from illness or injury, or disability from birth. In the restitution phase, patients are concerned with being ill but are aiming to get back to the normality that is being illness-free. The vocabulary in this phase is all around doctor and hospital appointments, scan and other test results, treatments and so on. So, in speech and language therapy terms, we could equate this with clients and carers focused on complete cure, complete restoration of communication skills to their premorbid level. Clients and carers might have this modernist restitution narrative as their only illness or disability narrative to date, and part of therapy might be the broaching of the fact that other stories of disability might have to be encountered.

In the chaos narrative, the client with an illness cannot envisage getting better. Their stories are disorganised and lack clarity; in fact, Frank refers to them as "anti-narratives" because the person in a state of chaos is unable to reflect and therefore to formalise thoughts into words or utterances. Again, attempting to align this with the world of speech and language therapy, clients with communication impairment who are in the chaos paradigm may not be in a state of readiness for therapy. Frank says that chaos stories are told "on the edge of speech…in the silences that speech cannot penetrate or illuminate" (p.101). This feels particularly pertinent for our clients for whom communication is a challenge, and leaves us as speech and language therapists asking the question: "Do I/am I able to listen to the chaos narrative of my clients and is this a part of my remit as therapist?"

The quest narrative is concerned with embracing the illness or disability, turning it into a force for good. This is perhaps exemplified by our past clients who go on to volunteer for charities such as the Stroke Association, who teach student speech and language therapists about what it is like to live with a communication impairment, or who become involved in patient advocacy in some way.

In terms of the therapeutic journey, it is hoped that clients will move into the quest narrative, able to resume their lives with perhaps an altered communication method but able to derive meaning and purpose again.

Mundle (2011) cites the narrative typologies of restitution, chaos and quest to suggest that therapists working with people with aphasia are facilitating the healing movement from chaos to quest in a "dialogical hermeneutical process" by being the "communicative body" that "transcends the verbal… bodies commune in touch, in tone, in facial expression and gestural attitude, and in breath" (Frank, 1995, p.49). This concept is perhaps familiar to speech and language therapists working with people with aphasia in the form of total communication and supported conversation. Mundle (2011) asserts that the role of therapist is one of 'co-creator' who accompanies the patient or client as they journey through the chaos and into their quest story. Therapy then is a redemptive activity, moving the client from chaos to quest, and arguably a spiritual enterprise, empowering the client to rediscover purpose, meaning and connection.

Liminality: The space between

Our clients with acquired communication impairment can be viewed as living 'betwixt and between' (Turner, 1967): their lived experience is between life before communication impairment and living life successfully *with* a communication impairment. Perhaps the role of the speech and language therapist is to steer the individual through this liminal space, this 'shipwreck' of the chaos narrative (Frank, 1995), to their place of quest. As speech and language therapists, perhaps we are also in a liminal space, on the threshold of including the spiritual in our management of clients with communication impairment, fully embracing all three aspects of our tripartite clients.

Policy and the national context

Person-centred care and patient dignity are both key drivers currently in the NHS, particularly following the Francis Report (Francis, 2013). It seems that in the latter part of the last century and the early years of this one, basic human care and compassion for our clients had been subsumed in the modernist search for cure, resolution and restitution. The medical model reigned, with Frank's restitution narrative at its heart; we were used to technology and experts being able to fix problems. We were used to healthcare professionals taking our case history, not listening to our story. We were used to passively accepting advice, pills and therapy, not mutually agreeing achievable goals.

Now in these postmodern times, we have come to recognise the responsibility and power we have over our own illnesses and lives, and that our therapy clients are the experts in their condition. As speech and language therapists we are to accompany them on their illness/disability journey in the role of facilitative travelling companion. Crucial to this model is an acceptance of the whole person, body, mind and spirit and a rejection of the hegemonic 'doctor knows best' mindset.

This shift in attitude is reflected in other key policies, including the NICE guidelines on end-of-life care (NICE, 2011) and the NHS National Service Framework for long-term conditions (DH, 2005), which both emphasise holism.

The World Health Organisation Quality of Life – Spirituality Religion and Personal Beliefs Group (WHOQOL-SRPB Group, 2006) identified these seven facets of spirituality:

- Spiritual connection
- Meaning and purpose in life
- Experiences of awe and wonder
- Wholeness and integration
- Spiritual strength
- Inner peace, hope and optimism
- Faith.

It is not only useful to regard spirituality in this manner in terms of finding a definition of sorts, but the fact that the WHO group exists reflects the fact that the organisation itself is concerned with spirituality, and considers it important enough to merit discussion in relation to healthcare.

Spirituality and other healthcare professionals

Occupational therapists seem to have travelled much further than the other therapies along the road of inclusion (or not) in their clinical work of issues relating to spirituality. In their conference of 2004, occupational therapists drew up a definition of spirituality:

> Spirituality can be defined as the search for meaning and purpose in life, which may or may not be related to a belief in God or some form of higher power. For those with no conception of supernatural belief, spirituality may relate to the notion of a motivating life force, which involves an integration of the dimensions of mind, body and spirit. This personal belief or faith also shapes an individual's

perspective on the world and is expressed in the way that he or she lives life. Therefore, spirituality is experienced through connectedness to God/a higher being, and/or by one's relationship with self, others or nature (Johnston and Mayers, 2005).

Because occupational therapy is inherently interested in the integration of all facets of the client in occupation, it makes intuitive sense that spirituality be included in models of occupation, and indeed it is, such as in the Canadian Model of Occupational Performance (CAOT, 1997). In fact, not only is spirituality included in the model, it is at the very centre of it, surrounded by other personal facets of the human condition such as the physical, cognitive and affective.

Kang (2003), another occupational therapist this time in Australia, has produced a new practice framework which she calls the "psychospiritual integration frame of reference for occupational therapy". She discusses the fact that spirituality encompasses centredness, connectedness, transcendence and meaning, and how these aspects of our clients can sometimes be neglected by healthcare professionals. Her framework therefore aims to encourage occupational therapists to engage with the spiritual facet of their clients in a systematic way.

No such integration of spirituality into the frameworks and practices of speech and language therapy seems to have occurred to date. In the US, a review of the literature revealed a convention presentation entitled "Exploring the role of spirituality in professional practice" (Spillers et al., 2009), given at a conference of the American Speech-Language-Hearing Association (ASHA) in New Orleans. In this study, speech and language therapy clients (both adults and children), clinicians and student speech and language therapy practitioners were interviewed, to obtain qualitative comments, and given a Likert-scale questionnaire to complete. Questions under consideration included, "What is spirituality?" "Is it the role of the speech and language therapist to discuss spirituality with their clients?" and "Should spirituality be included in speech and language therapy pre-registration curricula?". Interestingly, although over 80% of adult speech and language therapy clients stated that it was appropriate for speech and language therapists to address spirituality within their caring remit, and 92% of the adult clients reported that spirituality played an average to very large role in adjustment to their communication impairment, only 35% of the practising speech and language therapists felt that it was appropriate for them to address spirituality in their clinical practice. It seems, from this albeit limited example, that there is a marked disconnect between what clients feel is part of the speech and language therapist's role in regards to spirituality and what speech and language therapists themselves feel. Interestingly, 65% of speech and language therapy student practitioners were open to inclusion of spiritualty in the pre-registration speech and language therapy curricula.

There is no mention of spirituality in either the ASHA (2007), nor the Speech Pathology Australia (SPA) (2003) scope of practice documents. In the United Kingdom, the term 'spirituality' does not appear in either Communicating Quality 3 (RCSLT, 2006), nor in the RCSLT Clinical Guidelines (RCSLT, 2005).

Working together

If we acknowledge that holistic care implies care of all facets of the human condition – including spirituality – is it not incumbent upon the whole multidisciplinary team around a client to work together to ensure spiritual needs are met? I once met a chaplain who had worked previously in a stroke unit. He candidly confessed to avoiding patients with aphasia, because of the enormous difficulty of talking to – and therefore ministering to – people with limited communicative abilities. Perhaps as speech and language therapists with our expertise in facilitating communication, we are the best-placed healthcare professional in the team to empower our colleagues to communicate effectively with patients. Perhaps our remit should include facilitating spiritual conversations between client and chaplain, or training chaplains in best practice in terms of communicating with people with speech/language impairment.

In summary, spirituality is increasingly becoming an area of focus for healthcare professionals. It seems that the spiritual dimension of our clients should be an area that concerns our management of clients with illness or disability, if the whole person is to be considered and if therapy is to be construed as transformative and co-creational. In the post-Francis era of the six Cs (care, compassion, competence, communication, courage, commitment) (Francis, 2013), healthcare professionals should be encouraged and facilitated to embrace new ways of promoting dignity and real – not tokenistic – person-centred care. Nurses have thus far led the way in including the spiritual dimension within their curricula and work ethos. In terms of the therapies, occupational therapists have devised, and incorporated into their practice, models of psychospiritual care (Kang, 2003). Speech and language therapists have thus far not included the spiritual in their pre-registration curricula, nor in their day-to-day management of clients. Despite this, speech and language therapists are often in the unique and privileged position of having time and space to communicate with their clients with communication impairment, and are therefore well-placed to facilitate expressions of spirituality, in the pursuit of the quest narrative (Frank, 1995).

References

Baldacchino, D. (2008) Spiritual care: Is it the nurse's role? *Spirituality and Health International*, 9, 270–284.

Bash, A. (2004) Spirituality: The emperor's new clothes? *Journal of Clinical Nursing*, 13, 11–16.

Canadian Association of Occupational Therapists (CAOT) (1997) *Enabling Occupation: An Occupational Therapy Perspective*. Ottawa: CAOT Publications.

Cobb, M., Puchalski, C. & Rumbold, B. (2012) *Oxford Textbook of Spirituality in Healthcare*. Oxford: Oxford University Press.

Cruice, M., Worrall, L., Hickson, L. & Murison, R. (2003) Finding a focus for quality or life with aphasia: Social and emotional health, and psychological well-being. *Aphasiology*, 17(4), 333–353.

Duchan, J. (2001) *A History of Speech-Language Pathology*. Available online at www.acsu.buffalo.edu

Department of Health (2005) *National Service Framework for Long-term Conditions*. DH Publications.

Ellis-Hill, C. & Horn, S. (2000) Change to identity and self-concept: A new theoretical approach to recovery following stroke. *Clinical Rehabilitation*,14, 279–287.

Francis, R. (2013) *Report of the Mid Staffordshire NHS Foundation Trust Public Inquiry*. London: HMSO.

Frank, A.W. (1995) *The Wounded Storyteller*. Chicago: The University of Chicago Press.

Frankl, V. (2011) *Man's Search for Ultimate Meaning*. London: Rider.

Greenstreet, W. (Ed.) (2006) *Integrating Spirituality in Health and Social Care: Perspectives and Practical Approaches*. Oxford: Radcliffe.

Hilari, K., Wiggins, R., Roy, P., Byng, S. & Smith, S. (2003) Predictors of health-related quality-of life (HRQL) in people with chronic aphasia. *Aphasiology*, 17(4), 365–381.

Johnston, D. & Mayers, C. (2005) Spirituality: A review of how occupational therapists acknowledge, assess and meet spiritual needs. *British Journal of Occupational Therapy*, 68(9), 386–392.

Kang, C. (2003) A psychospiritual integration frame of reference for occupational therapy. Part 1: Conceptual foundations. *Australian Occupational Therapy Journal*, 50, 92–103.

Kay, J., Lesser, R. & Coltheart, D.(1992) *The Psycholinguistic Assessment of Language Processing in Aphasia*. Hove: Psychology Press.

Koubel, G. & Bungay, H. (2008) *The Challenge of Person-centred Care*. Basingstoke: Palgrave Macmillan.

Kvale, S. & Brinkmann, S. (2009) *InterViews. Learning the Craft of Qualitative Interviewing*. London: Sage.

Mackenzie, C., Muir, M. & Allen, C. (2010) Non-speech oromotor exercise use in acquired dysarthria management: Regimes and rationales. *International Journal of Language and Communication Disorders*, 45(6), 617–629.

Maslow, A.H. (1954) *Motivation and Personality*. New York: Longman.

McSherry, W. & Cash, K. (2004) The language of spirituality: An emerging taxonomy. *International Journal of Nursing Studies*, 41, 151–161.

McSherry, W., Cash, K. & Ross, L. (2004) Meaning of spirituality: Implications for nursing practice. *Journal of Clinical Nursing*, 13, 934–941.

McSherry, W. & Ross, L. (Eds) (2010) *Spiritual Assessment in Healthcare Practice*. Keswick: M and K Publishing.

Mundle, R. (2011) O word that I lack! Silence, speech and communicative bodies in the rehabilitation (and redemption) of stroke patients with expressive aphasia. *Journal of Religion, Disability and Health*, 15(3), 221–240.

NICE (2011) *Quality Standard for End-of-life Care for Adults*. http://www.nice.org.uk/guidance/QS13.

Potter, S. (1882) *Speech and its Defects. Considered Physiologically, Pathologically, Historically and Remedially*. Philadelphia, PA: P. Blakiston, Son & Co.

Spillers, C.S., Bongard, C., Deplazes, K.A., Gerard, J. & Narveson, R. (2009) *Exploring the Role of Spirituality in Professional Practice*. http://search.asha.org/default.aspx?q=spirituality

Swinburn, K., Porter, G. & Howard, D. (2004) *The Comprehensive Aphasia Test*. Hove: Psychology Press.

Turner, V. (1967). Betwixt and between: The liminal period in rites de passage. In V. Turner (Ed.) *The Forest of Symbols: Aspects of Ndembu Ritual*. New York: Cornell University Press.

Vargha-Khadem, F., Carr, L.J., Isaacs, E., Brett, E., Adams, C. & Mishkin, M. (1997) Onset of speech after left hemispherectomy in a nine year old boy. *Brain*, 120, 159–182.

World Health Organisation Quality of Life Spirituality Religion and Personal Beliefs (WHOQOL-SRPB) Group (2006) A cross-cultural study of spirituality, religion, and personal beliefs as components of quality of life. *Social Science and Medicine*, 62, 1486–1497.

7 Cultural and linguistic diversity issues in the profession

Jane Stokes

The lack of cultural and linguistic diversity within the speech and language therapy profession has been discussed and debated for over 25 years ,and although small changes have occurred in the UK it is still the case that the majority of speech and language therapists are white, female and monolingual. Although many clients accessing speech and language therapy services speak languages other than English, the approaches used in assessment and intervention draw largely on knowledge based on English, with scant information on other languages available to speech and language therapists. This chapter discusses issues that have often been swept under the collective professional carpet with reference to the approaches used by speech and language therapists when addressing important linguistic and cultural differences between them and the people they work with/for. The chapter reflects on concepts of cultural competence, cultural confidence and considers the inclusion of these in pre-registration education and continuing professional education.

Challenges for individual practitioners

When a child from a Cantonese-speaking family is diagnosed by a monolingual, English-speaking speech and language therapist as having specific language impairment (SLI) it is instructive to explore how this diagnosis has come about. Specific language impairment, or SLI, is typically a diagnosis of exclusion, based on a mismatch between verbal and non-verbal abilities, differences in the process of acquiring language in comparison with other children of same age, in the absence of developmental delay or hearing impairment (Bishop, 2001). This diagnosis when given for an English-speaking child has usually been arrived at by a mixture of developmental information, discussions with parents or carers, results of formal and informal assessments, consultation with educational staff and psychologists, and comparison with other English-speaking children of the same age.

Standardised tests are used for English-speaking children, but there are almost no standardised tests available for the most commonly-spoken community languages in the UK. In the case of the Cantonese-speaking child given a diagnosis, how has the child's first language been assessed? Has there actually been an assessment of the child's first language? Using what kinds of assessment? Has the therapist picked up the difference between code switching and confusion between languages? Has the therapist received training in the identification of SLI in bilingual children? Is he/she comfortable with the diagnosis? Has an interpreter or bilingual co-worker been involved in the assessment? Without a detailed knowledge of the stages of language development and knowledge of the effects of bilingualism on language development, the speech and language therapist has little to draw on in making such a diagnosis. At best, a diagnosis of SLI in a bilingual child is likely to be not much more than an informed guess. Speech and language therapists are right to feel uncertain when asked to make a diagnosis of this kind. Why is this still the case, 30 years after UK speech and language therapists established a special interest group to explore issues around bilingualism in order to address just such uncertainties?

Speech and language therapists in the UK report a range of responses to the challenge of working with families who do not share the same language as the therapist. Stokes (2000) found that therapists reported fear, anxiety, lack of confidence, and lack of knowledge of other languages. These hampered the therapists' ability to work with confidence in a culturally diverse population. Various US studies report on this lack of confidence of speech and language therapists when working with culturally and linguistically diverse clients (Kritikos, 2003; Hammer et al., 2004.) Chiuri (2012) reported that half the speech-language pathologists surveyed as part of her Ph.D. thesis did not feel confident in assessing clients from other linguistic backgrounds to their own, even with the aid of other personnel. Guiberson and Atkins (2012) surveyed speech and language therapists in Colorado and found a number of challenges associated with working with linguistic minority clients. These included a lack of ability to speak the client's language, lack of knowledge of developmental stages, lack of research, and a lack of interpreters. Kimble (2013) reported that most speech-language pathologists in a study of 192 professionals in the USA were uncomfortable assessing English language learners or limited English-proficient students and that years of experience were not significant in increasing comfort levels in working with such clients. She feels that this is due to ineffective pre-service education and lack of ongoing professional development.

Addressing the monolingualism of the profession

Despite the fact that these issues have been discussed in the profession for some time, there is still considerable concern that practitioners are poorly equipped and supported to work with culturally and linguistically diverse populations. Kayser in Lubinski and Hudson (2013) talks about the dearth of professionals from culturally and linguistically diverse backgrounds to meet the growing needs of these populations. We need professionals who understand cultural differences and who speak languages other than English (Hammer, 2011). Within speech and language therapy there is still a mismatch between "... the linguistic homogeneity of the...profession and the linguistic diversity of its clientele" (Caesar and Kohler, 2007, p.198). One possible solution might be to increase the numbers of people speaking relevant community languages in the profession of speech and language therapy. With a more culturally and linguistically diverse workforce, the anxieties and difficulties expressed by speech and language therapists in working with diverse populations might diminish. There are no readily available figures of speech and language therapists speaking community languages in the UK but there are some figures relating to ethnic origin. Care must obviously be taken not to equate ethnic origin with ability to speak minority languages. The UK charity Parity (www.parity-org.uk), which campaigns for equal rights, prepared a report in 2013 looking at the gender and ethnic breakdown of UK speech and language therapists. It quotes statistics from 2010 gathered by the Health and Care Professionals Council (HCPC), the registration body for speech and language therapists. These state that 92% of registrants were white with 2% identifying themselves as other, and less than 1% as Chinese. These compare with figures from the Royal College of Speech and Language Therapists (RCSLT) in 2002 which stated that 98.5% of speech and language therapists were white European in comparison to 1.5% of therapists who were recorded as other (RCSLT, 2002). Although the demography has changed somewhat since the figures were collected in 2002, in the UK speech and language therapy is still overwhelmingly a profession made up of people from white British backgrounds, many of whom speak English only. If therapists do speak languages other than English these are frequently not the languages represented on their caseload. In the USA, 7% of ASHA members identify themselves as bilingual or bicultural and 95% of school speech-language pathologists in the USA are white (ASHA, 2008). As long ago as 1985, ASHA developed a position statement and strategy for increasing the number of speech-language pathologists from culturally and linguistically diverse backgrounds. The RCSLT published a report on increasing diversity in the profession in 2002 (Thanki, 2002) but there has been little discernible corresponding action by the NHS, the profession's largest employer. There have been a few attempts at widening the diversity of recruitment of speech and language therapy students in the UK, (Madhani, 2004), but no coherent strategy across the universities.

Madhani (2004) discusses the issues in attracting students from minority ethnic communities to train as speech and language therapists. She points out that decisions about careers are often socially and culturally embedded, with parents and wider family involved in such decisions. Admissions procedures should be carefully scrutinised to ensure that there are no hidden discrimination factors. Greenwood, Wright and Bithell (2006) found that a possible explanation for the under-representation of minority ethnic students on speech and language therapy courses was a lack of awareness of the scientific nature of the career and its status as a degree profession.

Pre-registration training on cultural and linguistic diversity

While the RCSLT curriculum guidelines (2010) state that universities should include bilingualism in their teaching of speech and language therapy students, there is limited information given about what exactly should be covered. Lubinski and Matteliano (2008) provide a useful guide to teaching on cultural diversity within the curricula for educating speech and language therapists. They discuss the fact that curricula are already overloaded and argue not for separate courses on cultural competency but to incorporate this into existing courses. They feel that teaching on cultural competency and linguistic diversity should be integrated across the curriculum rather than constitute a separate module. This is in line with recommendations made by the UK Special Interest Group on Bilingualism (RCSLT, 1999); (RCSLT, 2002 available at www.londonsigbilingualism.co.uk/uniguide.html). According to Madhani (2004) "bilingualism and multilingualism can no longer be treated as an optional subject area" (p.13). Lubinski and Matteliano (2008) also talk about the need to acknowledge the fact that one's own biases and belief systems may have an impact on the provision of service; this could be more strongly highlighted in UK education of speech and language therapists. There is an important role for discussion of cultural awareness, cultural sensitivity and a place for self-assessment tools such as those available in the USA for example, the Cultural Values Questionnaire (Luckman, 2000). With an emphasis on including development of one's own cultural awareness, any teaching on reflective practice should incorporate this area.

Continuing professional development

Despite a recognition that there are problems, no coherent strategy or policy in the UK has been developed to address the difficulties expressed by speech and language therapists working with families from culturally and linguistically diverse communities. In the UK, the RCSLT has guidelines for best practice with this population (2007) but there is continuing concern in both the UK and the USA that therapists lack the appropriate knowledge and confidence.

There are limited opportunities for speech and language therapists to develop their knowledge of bilingualism. This was highlighted by Winter (1999) who discusses both over- and under-representation of bilingual clients relative to the populations served. She also discusses the fact that intervention models are based on white, middle-class monolingual cultures. The situation has not changed much since her important work. In the USA, there are three specific university courses on bilingual speech-language pathology. In the UK, there is an e-learning module available to members of the RCSLT. Although excellent, this is just a start.

The challenges facing the profession have been outlined by Mennen and Stansfield (2006): limited education on multilingual and multicultural issues, monolingual bias in research on speech and language therapy, lack of multilingual practitioners, scarcity of relevant resources and assessments and limited awareness by managers of the issues involved in working with linguistically diverse populations. The fundamental challenge, Mennen and Stansfield (2006) report, is the requirement for speech and language therapists to provide an equitable service in this context. Stow and Dodd (2003) also detail the factors that hinder the provision of an equitable service: the limitations in pre-registration education, training and recognition of bilingual co-workers, inappropriate assessment and intervention materials, and the paucity of relevant research.

Mennen and Stansfield (2006) conclude that the profession still has "some way to go towards providing an equitable service to multilingual children" (p.41), although they do make the point that the larger the population of minority language speakers, the more equitable the service appears to be.

Service provision

As far back as 1999, Winter found that 59% of therapists who work with children have at least one bilingual child on their caseload (Winter, 1999). This number is likely to have changed since then but there has been no recent published data of the number of bilingual children on the caseloads of UK speech and language therapists, and there are considerable difficulties in obtaining this information (Stow and Dodd, 2003). Mennen and Stansfield (2006) report on the inadequacy of recorded information on the linguistic breakdown of caseloads. Different services accord different levels of importance to recording such information and this makes planning of services more difficult.

Specialist posts in bilingualism were created during the 1980s and 1990s as the profession realised that there was a need to develop knowledge, resources and support for speech and language therapists working with diverse communities. With recent reorganisations, these specialist posts in bilingualism are being cut and bilingual co-workers – a model pioneered in several teams during the early 1980s – are now rare within speech and language therapy. Access to interpreting services is good in some areas but limited in others. Over ten years since Stow and Dodd (2003) made this point, there is still plenty of work to do to provide an equitable service.

In addition to addressing issues of service provision, some of which we can influence but some of which are vulnerable to economic and political influences that are bigger than just our profession, we could start to look in more detail at providing opportunities for practising speech and language therapists to engage in reflective activities relating to linguistic and cultural diversity. Given the lack of diversity and the slow rate of change, we need to consider putting systems in place to giving speech and language therapists protected time for reflective practice focusing on this issue. We can learn much from approaches to developing cultural awareness used in other countries and in other professions. There may in some organisations be mandatory training on cultural awareness but if staff are required to attend such courses, it can lead to resistance or superficial participation (Papadopoulos, 2003).

Cultural awareness, cultural competence

It is useful to understand some of the terms used in cultural awareness training. These concepts may have relevance for us as a profession and can stimulate reflection not only in students but also in practising clinicians. The introduction of issues related to cultural awareness could play an important part in regular supervision, discussion in teams, in-service training and team strategic planning events.

Griffer and Perlis (2007) describe the concept of cultural intelligence or CQ. Drawing on work by van Dyne, Ang and Koh (2009), they define CQ as comprising four components. The first is strategy, where individuals make sense of their own culturally diverse experiences, modifying their perceptions if these do not fit with their own expectations. The second is knowledge, where individuals learn about differences and similarities between cultures. The third is motivation, which relates to the individual's interest in learning, functioning and interacting within different cultural contexts, and the fourth is behaviour, which involves the ability to develop flexibility and adaptability in responding to people from diverse cultural backgrounds.

Griffer and Perlis (2007) also talk about the fact that the development of cultural intelligence begins with a study of self and the awareness that everyone has what they call a "multi-perspective identity". These perspectives are defined as those "characteristics of our identity that enable each individual to view reality through specific perspectives based upon ability, age, ethnicity, gender, race, religion, sexual orientation and socioeconomic class" (Perlis, 2001, p.11). Perhaps more time should be devoted in pre-registration education and in continuous professional education to exploring these aspects of our professional identity. Students and practising clinicians could be encouraged to reflect on their own identity or identities and what has shaped them. Tervalon and Murray-Garcia (1998) consider cultural competence as being a developmental process, requiring ongoing personal reflection, admission of limits and acquisition of knowledge. They discuss the development of what they call cultural humility. As well as reflecting on why they want to be speech and language therapists (see Chapter 9), they could consider what their cultural influences have been, how their own perspectives on other cultural groups have been shaped and developed. Everyone has a culture – this is not a term reserved for individuals of certain racial or cultural groups. It is useful for students and qualified practitioners to consider how they would describe their own culture, and how their own cultural background affects the way that they engage in clinical activity. It may be uncomfortable to look at these issues as there may be feelings that one has a different privileged position to those with whom we work, because of inequities of cultural and linguistic capital. Skilled supervision can be a place to help unpack some of these feelings (Chapter 3). Ryde (2009), disturbed by the lack of diversity in the helping professions, researched the nature of whiteness and how it impacts on helping relationships. She proposes that white people in the helping professions should explore their own racial and cultural identity. She suggests that unacknowledged advantages of being white may result in feelings of guilt or shame that are not addressed in the helping professions. She makes the insightful point that white people do not generally consider themselves as having a race, and feels that reflecting on this is a starting point for understanding ourselves in a political and social context. The unspoken power differences between people from western and non-western backgrounds are rarely discussed in speech and language therapy in the UK. Many individuals that we work with may come from subcultures or contra-cultures according to Griffer and Perlis (2007). These individuals may perceive the speech-language pathologist as one who cannot understand their world view and therefore cannot help them.

In addition to the concept of cultural intelligence, a number of other terms are used, often interchangeably. Terms such as cultural awareness, cultural sensitivity and cultural competence have been explored in relation to health and education professions. O'Hagan (2001) defines cultural competence as the ability to "maximise sensitivity and minimize insensitivity in the service of culturally diverse communities" (p.235). Papadopoulos (2003) describes the development of a model for conceptualising and measuring cultural competence in nursing professions; this has not been specifically applied to speech and language therapy, although it has great relevance for all health professions. It involves the different components of cultural awareness, cultural knowledge and cultural sensitivity and gives pointers as to how these can be developed. In 2008, the London Deanery, which provided support on professional development for doctors in the UK before it was reorganised, reviewed the literature on cultural competence and found there was misunderstanding and confusion about the term and that professional development in this area was variable and not prioritised (http://www.londondeanery.ac.uk/var/equality-diversity/cultural-competence/what-is-cultural-competence).

The London Special Interest Group on Bilingualism, which acts as a professional learning community for speech and language therapists in London, has published a number of useful documents on its website (www.

londonsigbilingualism.co.uk) which provide a resource for individuals and teams exploring cultural competence. In the USA, ASHA has developed a cultural competence checklist. This gives a structure for looking at the policies of one's organisation and a tool for self-assessment of cultural competence. But for all these documents, the practising speech and language therapist has to go looking for them. The development of cultural competence is not accorded high priority in continuous professional development. It might be useful to consider the ways in which this area could be given greater emphasis through, for example, the log of continuous professional development provided by the RCSLT or in staff appraisals. There should be increased opportunities for exploring the links between cultural identity and health, cultural identity and disability and an appreciation of how societal and organisational structures reflect and influence culture.

Part of the problem is in the difficulty of measuring cultural competence. There is also limited evidence that training on it is effective (Papadopoulos, 2003). It is perhaps best viewed not as a competency to be achieved but as a developmental and evolving period of growth. Battle (2000) described cultural competence as "a process through which one develops an understanding of self, while developing the ability to develop responsive, reciprocal, and respectful relationships with others" (p.19). In this way, this process should be just an extension of the reflective practice that we all are encouraged to engage in as healthcare practitioners. When we see cultural competence in this light, it should simply reflect best practice. Is there therefore such a problem? Yes, because without an explicit focus on the importance of reflecting on one's own culture and belief systems, the process of developing cultural competence is at risk of becoming nonspecific and watered down. There could be more developed guidance and support for speech and language therapists exploring their own identity. It should be an integral part of both pre-registration education and post-qualification education

An increase in therapists' confidence in working with culturally and linguistically diverse communities will also come as we gain more knowledge and disseminate more information about other languages. McLeod, Verdon and Bowen (2013) have done some excellent work in drawing together information on speech sound disorders in different languages – just such information is what speech and language therapists require to build their awareness and increase their knowledge. Their position paper also highlights the key issues and challenges and introduces the concept of cultural safety, drawing on earlier work by Williams (1999) who defined a culturally safe health/

education environment as "where there is no assault, challenge or denial of their identity, of who they are and what they need. It is about shared respect, shared meaning, shared knowledge and experience, of learning together with dignity, and truly listening" (p.213).

Addressing the challenges

We have so far explored the wider issues relating to cultural competence and many lessons can be learned from work carried out with other professional groups. For speech and language therapy practice in particular there are a number of challenges. There is an imperative for managers of speech and language therapy to address the feelings of fear, inadequacy, anxiety, and loss of control described by therapists when working with culturally and linguistically diverse communities (Stokes, 2000). Newly-appointed therapists can be supported by an induction period to include observation of more experienced colleagues working with interpreters or bilingual co-workers and regular opportunities in individual supervision sessions for case discussion, and reflections on their own cultural competence. Appraisal targets could include development of cultural awareness, study time on relevant topics. Team joint work could include developing systems for accurate recording and collection of information about different linguistic groups served, jointly prepared advice for staff working, and a thorough examination of each stage of the therapy process to check potential areas of cultural and linguistic bias. There must be a recognition that, in order to develop one's cultural competence, there needs to be allocated time for training, supervision and support.

In order to gain confidence in the assessment and intervention processes, there needs to be training both at pre-registration and post-qualification levels about the challenges associated with working across languages. Caesar and Kohler (2007) found a continued reliance on formal standardised approaches to assessment despite the fact that the majority of assessments have been standardised on English, and guidance explicitly cautions against this. The New Reynell Developmental Language Scales (2011) have a useful multilingual toolkit to guide the assessment of children with languages other than English. Alternative approaches to the use of standardised assessment need to be considered: language sampling and analysis, dynamic assessment, curriculum-based approaches. The International Association of Logopaedics and Phoniatrics (IALP) (www.ialp.info) has published guidelines on working with linguistically diverse communities, the RCSLT has guidelines for best practice (2007) and ASHA has a wealth of useful information related to this on their website, www.asha.org.

Stokes and Madhani (in press) describe different approaches to assessment when one does not share the language of the family, emphasising partnership with the family, and the need to consider sociocultural aspects of disability.

Intervention decisions must be made in conjunction with the families, drawing on sound evidence. Therapists need to be aware of the issues relating to advice on what language to use with a child, remaining respectful of the family's views while using best practice. Again, therapists should be allowed time and resources to keep up to date with recent literature on this (Guiberson and Atkins 2012; McLeod et al., 2013).

With the increase in diversity of the population and the relative cultural and linguistic homogeneity of the speech and language therapy profession, there is a need to develop our knowledge and our confidence. But an overarching imperative is to strengthen our frameworks for reflective practice that will ensure that our profession grows in its ability to provide an equitable service. The average white, English-speaking therapist will never have an encylopaedic knowledge of every language and cultural group he or she is likely to encounter in clinical practice. There will never be formal assessments available in all community languages represented on the caseload. There must therefore be:

(a) a commitment made by all therapists to their own professional development in this area

(b) provision of support and supervision specifically addressing issues of cultural identity, and

(c) an acknowledgement that we need to go beyond the narrow skills associated with linguistic and phonological analysis.

We need to be able to approach the culturally and linguistically diverse communities in which we work with an openness and respect, coupled with a willingness to learn. This self-awareness is, as O'Hagan (2001), says "the most important component in the knowledge base of culturally competent practice" (p.235).

References

American Speech-Language-Hearing Association (2008) *Schools Survey Report: Workforce and Work Conditions Trends 2000–2008*. Rockville, MD: Author.

Battle, D.E. (2000) Becoming a culturally competent clinician. *ASHA Special Interest Group 1: Perspectives on Language Learning and Education*, 7, 20–23.

Bishop, D. (2001) Genetic and environmental risks for specific language impairment in children. *Philosophical Transactions of the Royal Society of London Series B Biological Sciences*, 356, 369–380.

Caesar, L. & Kohler, P. (2007) The state of school-based bilingual assessment: Actual practice versus recommended guidelines. *Language, Speech, and Hearing Services in Schools*, 38(3), 190–200.

Chiuri, G. (2012) Speech Language Pathologists' Perceptions of Services to Children from Culturally and Linguistically Diverse Backgrounds. Ph.D. dissertation available at https://beardocs.baylor.edu:8443/xmlui/handle/2104/8414

Greenwood, N., Wright, J. & Bithell, C. (2006) Perceptions of speech and language therapy amongst UK school and college students: Implications for recruitment. *International Journal of Language and Communication Disorders*, 41(1), 83–94.

Griffer, M. & Perlis, S. (2007) Developing cultural intelligence in pre-service speech-language pathologists and educators. *Communication Disorders Quarterly*, 29(1), 28–35.

Guiberson, M. & Atkins, J. (2012) Speech-language pathologists' preparation, practices and perspectives on serving culturally and linguistically diverse children. *Communication Disorders Quarterly*, 33(3), 169–180.

Hammer, C.S., Detwiler, J.S., Detwiler, J., Blood, G.W. & Qualls, C.D. (2004) Speech-language pathologists' training and confidence in serving Spanish-English bilingual children. *Journal of Communication Disorders*, 37, 91–108.

Hammer, C.S. (2011) Broadening our knowledge about diverse populations. *American Journal of Speech-Language Pathology*, 20, 71–72.

International Association of Logopaedics and Phoniatrics (IALP) *Recommendations for Working with Bilingual Children* (updated May 2011). http://www.ialp.info.

Kayser, H. (2013) Service delivery for culturally and linguistically diverse populations. In R. Lubinski,& M. Hudson (Eds) (2013) *Professional Issues in Speech-Language Pathology and Audiology*, 4th ed. New York: Delmar Engage.

Kimble, C. (2013) Speech-language pathologists' comfort levels in English language learner service delivery. *Communication Disorders Quarterly*, 35(1), 21–27.

Kritikos, E. (2003) Speech-language pathologists' beliefs about language assessment of bilingual/bicultural individuals. *American Journal of Speech-Language Pathology*, 12, 73–91.

Lubinski, R. & Hudson, M. (Eds) (2013) *Professional Issues in Speech-Language Pathology and Audiology*, 4th ed. New York: Delmar Engage.

Lubinski, R. & Matteliano, M.A. (2008) *A Guide to Cultural Competence in the Curriculum: Speech-Language Pathology*. Center for International Rehabilitation Research Information and Exchange. New York: Buffalo.

Luckman, J. (2000) *Transcultural Communication in Health Care*. Albany: Delmar.

Madhani, N. (2004) Attracting students from ethnic communities. RCSLT *Bulletin*, 623, 12–13.

McLeod, S., Verdon, S. & Bowen, C. (2013) International aspirations for speech-language pathologists' practice with multilingual children with speech sound disorders: Development of a position paper. *Journal of Communication Disorders*, 46, 375–387.

Mennen, I. & Stansfield, J. (2006) Speech and language therapy services to multilingual children in Scotland and England: A comparison of three cities. *Journal of Multilingual Communication Disorders*, 4(1), 23–44.

New Reynell Developmental Language Scales (2011) Gl Assessment. http://www.gl-assessment.co.uk

O'Hagan, K. (2001) *Cultural Competence in the Caring Professions*. London: Jessica Kingsley.

Papadopoulos, I. (2003) The Papadopoulos, Tilki and Taylor model for the development of cultural competence in nursing. *Journal of Health, Social and Environmental Issues*, 4(1), 5–7.

Parity (2013) Briefing Paper: Gender Balance in Public Sector Professions: Speech and Language Therapy. http://www.parity-uk.org

Perlis, S. (2001) *Sexual Orientation and Multiperspective Identity on a Small, Catholic Campus: An Analysis of the Cultural Climate and Multicultural Organizational Change*. Doctoral dissertation, Temple University, Philadelphia.

Royal College of Speech and Language Therapists (1999) *Teaching about Bilingualism and Linguistic Minority Clients in Speech and Language Therapy Courses*. London: RCSLT.

Royal College of Speech and Language Therapists (2002) *Developing a Diversity Strategy*. London: RCSLT.

Royal College of Speech and Language Therapists (2007) *Good Practice for Speech and Language Therapists Working with Clients from Linguistic Minority Communities*. London: RCSLT.

Royal College of Speech and Language Therapists (2010) *Guidelines for Pre-registration Speech and Language Therapy Courses in the UK*. London: RCSLT.

Ryde, M. (2009) *Being White in the Helping Professions*. London: Jessica Kingsley.

Stokes, J. (2000) Strategies for Working with Clients from Multilingual Backgrounds. Paper presented at International Association of Logopaedics and Phoniatrics, 2nd International Symposium of Communication Disorders in Multilingual Populations, South Africa.

Stokes, J. & Madhani, N. (in press) Perspectives on working with preschool children from Panjabi, Gujarati, and Bengali speaking families. In J. Patterson & B. Rodriguez (in press). *Multilingual Perspectives on Child Language Disorders*. Bristol: Multilingual Matters.

Stow C. & Dodd, B. (2003) Providing an equitable service to children in the UK: A review. *International Journal of Language and Communication Disorders*, 38, 351–377.

Tervalon, M. & Murray-Garcia, J. (1998). Cultural humility versus cultural competence: A critical distinction in defining physician training outcomes in multicultural education. *Journal of Health Care for the Poor and Underserved*, 9(2), 117–124.

Thanki, M. (2002) *'White Women Only'. The Challenge for Change*. RCSLT Diversity Strategy Report. London: RCSLT.

Van Dyne, L., Ang, S. & Koh, C. (2009) Cultural intelligence: Measurement and scale development. In M.A. Moodian (Ed.) *Contemporary Leadership and Inter-cultural Competence: Exploring the Cross-Cultural Dynamics within Organizations*. Thousand Oaks: Sage.

Williams, R. (1999) Cultural safety: What does it mean for our work practice? *Australian and New Zealand Journal of Public Health*, 23(2), 213–214.

Winter, K. (1999) Speech and language therapy provision for bilingual children: Aspects of the current service. *International Journal of Language and Communication Disorders*, 34, 85–98.

8 Speech and language therapy and gender

Chris Markham and Catherine Neal

Introduction

Gender bias in the service sector, particularly in 'caring' and 'empathic' professions, such as nursing, teaching and speech and language therapy, is a situation that has been discussed in the professional and academic literature for several years. Riddell and Tett (2010) suggest that conventional, social representations of masculinity prohibit men from entering such professions. Indeed, Wilson (1998) reported that 79 percent of NHS employees were women, despite numerous policy changes and even the Sex Discrimination Act HMSO, 1975), which opened to men new professional opportunities, such as midwifery (Miers, 2000).

Speech and language therapy is concerned with an individual's communication and swallowing (Norton, 2013). People of all ethnicities, ages and genders require support and work with speech and language therapists, yet there is a gender and cultural bias to the demography of the profession. In particular, male speech and language therapists are under-represented (Greenwood, Wright and Bithell, 2006). In many ways this is not dissimilar to the demographic characteristics of the multidisciplinary teams that speech and language therapists work within, including allied health professions, nursing and teaching. The degree of under-representation is less marked in these professions, however, than in speech and language therapy. Indeed, data from the Health and Care Professions Council have suggested that only 2.5 percent of speech and language therapy registrants are male (McKinson, 2007). This figure is consistent with trends over time and leads to numerous questions, including what deters men from entering speech and language therapy as a profession or, alternatively, what inspires (principally) women to go into the profession.

This chapter examines gender and its role within the profession of speech and language therapy. It explores the influence of gender and employment roles more broadly within our culture and then focuses specifically on the field of speech and language therapy. The second part of the chapter presents some preliminary research data concerning gender and the experience of men training and working as a speech and language therapists.

Gender

The term 'gender' was discussed in the 1960s by psychiatrist Robert Stoller, and is now referred to as a learnt behaviour, as opposed to 'sex', which is our biological identity (Holmes, 2007). Society and its 'mores' shape the way males and females behave and the decisions they make, including within their careers. When referring to masculinity, many are referring to 'hegemonic masculinity'. Fuller (1996) describes five 'core attributes': possession of work or money; heterosexuality; non-femininity; manliness; denial of vulnerability; and emotion. If one of these attributes is missing, the male is no longer masculine and invites 'gender trouble' (Butler, 1990). In the context of hegemonic masculinity, then, it is incongruous for males to express feelings of vulnerability or to empathise with those experiencing it (Fuller, 1996).

Historically, women would work at home, looking after children and the home, whilst men engaged in paid work to provide financial support for the family. Indeed, during the 19th century, employment and social legislation concerning child labour encouraged the consolidation of this status quo. Increasingly, women maintained unpaid caring roles whilst men pursued improved working opportunities, leading to greater financial return to support their families (Holmes, 2009). Oakley (1972) refers to what 'mothers' do with their children and that 'mothers' should be the caregivers, excluding males from this role. Holmes (2009) argues that, if gender is learnt, ideas around what is masculine and feminine evolve and change over time.

Traditional occupations

According to the core attributes of hegemonic masculinity, a male will choose a career which generates a lot of money and power, have the opportunity to show strength, be it physical or intellectual, and avoid showing, or empathising with, vulnerable emotions (Lupton, 2000). Choices of GCSE subjects influence the choice of career made later in life; subjects chosen directly affect skills learnt for specific careers. The Office of the First Minister and Deputy First Minister, in Northern Ireland, found that gender differences are prominent with males choosing physics and chemistry, while females choose languages and biology at GCSE level (OFMDFM, 2011). Males are found to subsequently join courses such as engineering and computing when entering further education, while females choose health, social studies and languages, all of which include skills utilised in speech and language therapy (Wright and Kersner 2009). Thirty percent of females follow paths in health and education at university against 2.3 percent of males. It is unsurprising, therefore, that there were no male nursery nurses working between 2003 and 2011 (OFMDFM, 2011). According to the Office of National Statistics (ONS) (2013), 1.55 million people work for the National Health Service (NHS), of which three-quarters are female (Breitenbach, 2006). Within speech and language therapy, males make up 2.5 percent of speech and language therapists in the UK (McKinson, 2007).

According to the Equality and Human Rights Commission (2010), gender accounts for more differences in occupations than any other category. Also, there are more problems reported for gay men in occupations such as teaching, due to negative perceptions from the public, than heterosexuals. It is widely accepted for females to be in traditionally male industries but there is still stigma around males in traditionally female jobs. This may be why, when a male enters a female-dominated profession, they have been seen to behave in ways which express their hegemonic masculinity as a way of proving themselves (Lupton, 2000).

Males as criminals

In recent years, males have contributed to the greatest degree of criminal activity in the UK, with 25 percent of males having committed a crime (Ministry of Justice, 2010). In 2011/12 there were 5778 cases of sexual activity with a minor reported by the police, and 99 percent of the offenders were male (Ministry of Justice, Home Office & the Office for National Statistics, 2013). With such a disproportionate crime rate relating to gender, the public may mistrust males, especially when working with vulnerable people, which those with speech, language and communication needs tend to be.

Gender issues are not only confined to the field of speech and language therapy, but have been reported across all female-dominated professions. One example is primary school teaching. In 2003, nearly 90 percent of primary school teachers were female (Riddell and Tett, 2006). There is a paucity of literature concerning speech and language therapy, and therefore the search for literature was widened to include primary school teachers as well as nurses, to find their views on gender-related issues. Searches revealed more implications for males who work with children than adults, so this literature review will also focus on issues surrounding child–adult relations. Eight themes were produced from the article findings. These were: awareness, professional and personal interactions with speech and language therapists, salary, public perceptions, career progressions, safeguarding, isolation and personal interest.

Awareness

A pertinent finding from studies conducted with speech and language therapy students and professionals is a lack of awareness of the profession (Boyd and Hewlett, 2001; Byrne, 2007; Greenwood et al., 2006; Litosseliti and Leadbeater, 2012; McAllister and Neve, 2005). Boyd and Hewlett (2001) discovered that careers advisers for the students at school were "discouraging, unhelpful and vague" (p.170). In fact, one student reported that the careers adviser had tried to dissuade him from speech and language therapy by saying the skills acquired are non-transferable and that males would not progress within the profession.

However, interestingly, those in this study, who had been qualified for five to ten years, had received positive experiences with careers advisers. McAllister and Neve (2005) found support for the former, as the careers advisers they interviewed seemed to have little knowledge of the profession but stated that it is unfair to expect that they know about every profession in detail. They also admitted to directing males in other directions regarding the field of health because of their gender. These students were also persuaded by their peers to complete a degree that was seen as 'traditionally male'. One third of participants in the study conducted by Greenwood et al. (2006) claimed they had never heard of speech and language therapy and that they had no idea what a speech and language therapist does, the majority being male, although white participants were significantly more aware. Most students found information from university websites (Byrne, 2007), although some students claimed that when wanting to research the profession, finding information proved difficult (McAllister and Neve, 2005). Campaigns to educate the public via social media sites and other forms of media have been suggested (Litosseliti and Leadbeater, 2012), and more work experience opportunities would be a good way to encourage new students into the profession (McAllister and Neve, 2005).

Professional and personal interaction with speech and language therapy

Working in related professions, for example in health care or education settings, is a major factor in the decision to pursue speech and language therapy as very few participants joined a speech and language therapy course straight after school (Boyd and Hewlett, 2001; Byrne, 2007; McAllister and Neve, 2005). Byrne (2007) found that 69 percent of her participants had prior exposure to speech and language therapy and further noted that of those participants who had come straight from school, over 60 percent had parents in a health or education setting, which was usually the mother. Greenwood et al. (2006) also found that those who had a relative in health care work would be more inclined to consider speech and language therapy as a career. Some of the speech and language therapists reported that they had been given the opportunity to observe some therapy before settling upon the career (Litosseliti and Leadbeater, 2012; McAllister and Neve, 2005). However, the speech and language therapists they had been shadowing were family members. Personal interactions with a speech and language therapist, for example having relatives or close family friends who have received speech and language therapy, are found to positively influence a decision to follow the career (Byrne, 2007; Litosseliti and Leadbeater, 2012; McAllister and Neve, 2005). Byrne (2007) found had it not been for their first-hand experience with the relative receiving speech and language therapy, those individuals would not have known about what is involved and the potential outcomes of speech and language therapy, which were all described positively.

Salary

High-school careers advisers noted that males are more likely than females to desire a job with a high salary status (Litosseliti and Leadbeater, 2012) and suggested that many males in NHS careers are actually within lower salaried employment, an observation also reflected in Loan-Clarke et al. (2009). Loan-Clarke et al. (2009) also found that low pay, which does not match the responsibilities required for the job, contributes to reasons for leaving the NHS. Males have also reported that the remuneration in speech and language therapy was not sufficient to sustain the lifestyle they desired, for example supporting a growing family. Because of this, only two participants reported that they saw themselves still working as a speech and language therapist in the long-term future (McAllister and Neve, 2005). The college students from Greenwood et al.'s (2006) study reflect the careers adviser's observations, with 86 percent of males expressing high salary as an important factor for a degree choice. However, it is not stated exactly what 'high salary' means to the college student. It is also not stated whether the participants in these studies work for a government body (e.g., NHS) or whether some work in independent practices.

Career progression

Males have been reported to seek high-status employment roles. For example, male speech and language therapists working within education were reported to reach the highest position quickly so searched for jobs within management (McAllister and Neve, 2005). This is reflected in Litosseliti and Leadbeater's (2012) study, with one male speech and language therapist suggesting that males in managerial roles look after one another and tend to promote them more quickly than they do females. This has also been noted in research on primary school teachers (Cushman, 2010; Thornton and Bricheno, 2000). Cross and Bagilhole (2002) found that 100 percent of the male primary school teachers surveyed had sought promotion, whereas only 71 percent of females had.

When choosing a career, self-employment was an attractive factor, especially for males (Greenwood et al., 2006). In addition, career prospects were important for both males and females. Lack of career progression was stated as a reason for considering leaving speech and language therapy when working in the NHS (Loan-Clark et al., 2009) and by all the males in McAllister and Neve's (2005) study. Females often have a gap in their career for maternity leave and subsequent childcare responsibilities, which can retard career progression (Loan-Clarke et al., 2009). These could, therefore, be seen as incentives for males to join these professions.

Public perceptions

Speech and language therapy has been found to be associated with a negative public stigma (Byrne 2007; Greenwood et al., 2006; Litosseliti and Leadbeater, 2012; Loan-Clarke et al., 2009; McAllister and Neve, 2005). Litosseliti and

Leadbeater (2012) suggest that the words 'speech', 'language' and 'therapy' are all unconsciously associated with females by society, which discourages males. They suggest that a simple change of name could remedy this. The college students in Greenwood et al.'s (2006) study were aiming for a high prestige, scientific career and were unlikely to choose speech and language therapy. It was perceived that speech and language therapists 'play around' and that there is 'no seriousness to it' (p.92). Shockingly, this was reported as a view from within speech and language therapy itself (Litosseliti and Leadbeater, 2012). Primary school teachers have also been seen as 'glorified baby sitters' (p.205); the younger the children, the lower the status of the teacher (Thornton and Bricheno, 2000; Skelton, 2003). Indeed, some nurses and teachers choose not to disclose their profession because of fears that the public would look badly upon them and that people may question their sexuality. The latter was an important concern in Cross and Bagilhole's (2002) study, especially if the perception was from male peers from other professions. To overcome this, males suggested having pride in their work and that being assertive helps to keep a sense of 'being a man'. On the other hand, students currently studying speech and language therapy said that they chose the course because English and science are equally incorporated (Byrne, 2007). Byrne (2007) also reports only positive feedback from those who had experienced speech and language therapy passively, i.e., by watching a relative. This further suggests that it is the lack of knowledge of the work which may prevent some people from choosing the career.

Safeguarding

Males are made to feel more aware of issues around child abuse than females (Boyd and Hewlett, 2001; Cushman, 2010; Skelton, 2003). One speech and language therapist reported that he was asked to leave the door open when working alone with a child (Boyd and Hewlett, 2001). However, safeguarding is a greater influencing variable in primary school teachers than in speech and language therapy. This may be because the majority of speech and language therapists interviewed worked with adults rather than children, whereas primary school teachers work with young children every day.

In society, and usually from the parents' point of view, it is perceived as strange if a man wants to work with young children and especially children in the early years (Skelton, 2003). There is 'paranoia' around safeguarding (Cushman, 2005) and some primary school teachers find the rules around it frustrating because they had been encouraged to nurture pupils with hugs, while in practice this is frowned upon. Furthermore, many primary school teaching students have reported that they were constantly warned about physical contact, usually by female colleagues (Cushman, 2010). Indeed, some primary school teachers were made to feel so uncomfortable that they perceived no other choice but to leave the profession. Others had accepted this as the culture and some did not feel uncomfortable about the rules at all, believing it not to be an issue and saying that men naturally avoid hugging (Cross and Bagilhole, 2002). Furthermore, males also do not see that these perceptions will change in the future (Skelton, 2003).

Isolation

Typically, there will be only one or two males working within a team of females, which can leave males feeling isolated, vulnerable and sometimes wanting a role model (Boyd and Hewlett, 2001; Cross and Bagilhole, 2002; Cushman, 2005, 2010; Thornton and Bricheno, 2000). Boyd and Hewlett (2001) reported that just under a third of the male speech and language therapists interviewed reported concerns relating to isolation, due to females feeling threatened by them. Also, males felt as if they had to justify themselves as a trustworthy and qualified person. The same issue can be found with primary school teachers. For example, within the staff room, one male primary school teacher reported that women and men are interested in different conversation topics which leaves males craving more masculine conversation (Cushman, 2005). It seems that speech and language therapy educators can also exacerbate this issue. For example, in the same group of student speech and language therapists, the male was given a placement in a hospital, yet females were not (Litosseliti and Leadbeater, 2012), which could cause further isolation due to separation. Male primary school teachers reported being given the manual jobs within the school, such as lifting, by the females, and a feeling that the females send the naughtier children to the males to play a disciplinary role which adds extra pressure for them (Cushman, 2005).

Conversely, McAllister and Neve (2005) found that none of the speech and language therapy students in their study had been subject to any stereotyping from females. Also, 'banter' has been found to be a way around the gender differences. Then again, it was said that the males are usually the 'whipping boys' (Cross and Bagilhole, 2002, p.218). If males were to banter in the way females do, and use the females as the 'scapegoat', this could cause further concerns and possibly even escalate into a legal matter.

Personal interest

Despite stereotypical ideas to the contrary within the literature, it is evident from some research that the majority of males do not work in these fields for the salary or career structure alone; rather, it is because of a personal sense of helping others (Byrne, 2007; Loan-Clarke et al., 2009; McAllister and Neve, 2005). For example, males that have joined speech and language therapy courses report an awareness that salary might not be as high as their peers within other professions and that there may be limited opportunities for career progression (McAllister and Neve, 2005). Indeed, many males have agreed that it was the clinical role that attracted them to the profession, because of a desire to make an impact and positively contribute to service users lives (Byrne, 2007). Set against evidence such as this, though, are examples, such as Boyd and Hewlett's (2001) research, which suggest that gender stereotyping in speech and language therapy discourages men from pursuing a career that is regarded as a primarily a feminine occupation.

More broadly, this has been explained by the cultural expectations of 'men's' and 'women's' career aspirations. Within the nursing profession, Xu (2008) suggests that career progression is associated with males' attraction to elevated positions, higher wages, advanced technology and power. Xu (2008) argues that, even within nursing, men tend to work within clinical specialities involving greater healthcare technologies and that management posts are disproportionately populated by men rather than women. Indeed, Litosseliti and Leadbeater (2012) found that inequality within the speech and language therapy profession led to the 'glass escalator effect' (Williams, 1992, p.256, cited in Litosseliti and Leadbeater, 2012), where men's careers trajected into more senior roles disproportionately sooner than female counterparts.

In addition to explanations around status and salary, research has concluded that awareness of speech and language therapy as a profession is also a contributing factor in the low recruitment of male speech and language therapists. Greenwood et al. (2006) demonstrate that school- and college-aged males are less familiar with speech and language therapy than females and both males and females were unclear as to what speech and language therapists actually do. Furthermore, perceptions of salaries and status are misunderstood. Greenwood et al. (2006) discovered that the majority of young people involved in their study regarded speech and language therapists as being closely related to nurses and therefore earning the same or similar wages. Similarly, Litosseliti and Leadbeater's (2012) work suggests that male perceptions of wages of speech and language therapists are misinterpreted and many young males stated that they "want to be engineers or they want to earn lots of money and work in the city" (p.7). Again these perceptions can be found in other, related careers, such as teaching, where views of young, career seeking men demonstrated a shared perception that teaching as a profession involved low pay and social status (Riddell and Tett, 2010).

Furthermore, Whittock and Leonard (2003) suggest that fewer men pursue speech and language therapy due to their concerns regarding the potential reaction from family and friends, related to social expectations of masculinity. Indeed, this theme is explored further by Cross and Bagilhole's (2002) research with men in female-dominated professions, particularly in their observation of participants' responses that "nearly half actually conceal their occupation from their friends and the strangers they meet" (p.222). This relates to evidence regarding concerns about men working with children being suspicious (Skelton, 2003). Research by Cushman (2005) shows that men who consider employment in primary schools often reconsidered it, as they felt parents and colleagues would consider it inappropriate to teach young children, some even expressing suspicion of sexual perversity. For men, as Francis and Skelton (2001) cited in Cushman (2005) point out, moral panic about paedophilia may actually be a reason to deter men away from working with children.

Similarly, within 'caring' professions, a male role can be defined by stereotypical ideas of masculinity. Whittock and Leonard (2003) comment on how men are expected to do 'masculine work' such as managing aggressive patients and manual labour. Meadus and Twomey (2011) agreed with these results and their outcomes also showed that men perceived their professional roles defined by their gender and its perceived masculinity, describing an expectation that they would fulfil physical tasks, such as managing challenging behaviour (and restraint), in clinical care situations.

Dahlborg-Lyckhage and Pilhammar-Anderson (2009) showed that young peoples' interests are influenced by the media's portrayal of societal positions and behavioural characteristics that are typical of men and women. This research states that nurses lack power at an organisational level and that generally, in nursing, males and females stick with the 'status quo'. Meadus and Twomey (2011) agreed with these findings and expressed the public's understanding of nursing being a feminine role. They found that in modern society men and women are still assigned to clinical areas on placement, dependent on gender. For example, few men in their study were placed in maternity wards or other 'typically' feminine areas. Indeed, Whittock and Leonard's (2003) research suggests that men can feel excluded from gender-specific careers.

Recent research

Evidence from unpublished research reflects a number of the existing themes discussed so far. We have conducted qualitative interviews with male speech and language therapy students and both male and female therapists concerning their experiences and beliefs regarding gender and the speech and language profession. The themes within these findings reflect negative experiences of male students and therapists within the profession and established assumptions that men within caring professions seek higher status roles within management.

Interviews were conducted with two male speech and language therapy students and three male and two female clinicians. Interviews were open and utilised a minimum of prompts and probes, from topic guides aimed at illuminating the experiences and perceptions of research participants in order to contribute an additional perspective to our understanding of gender and the profession. This research took a qualitative design, using a thematic analysis to describe the data. Qualitative research was most likely to illuminate the participants' individual opinions and feelings, thereby yielding subjective findings, which could be interpreted and inform detailed explanations grounded in the participants' (male and female) experiences.

Given the paucity of males within the speech and language therapy student and professional populations, purposeful sampling of men was a challenge and, consequently, convenience sampling was employed to recruit male participants from the profession and the 2012–2013 UK student body. Convenience sampling was also used to recruit female speech and language therapist participants in order to provide an additional and alternative perspective.

The study utilised face-to-face, in-depth, semi-structured interviews. All interviews were conducted in university interview rooms and recorded on a digital voice recorder. Each interview began with an open-ended question or statement. Participants were encouraged to not stop talking until they had explored all their views on the topics raised. If participants 'realised' ideas they had not had before, they were encouraged to enter into a 'stream of consciousness' and to 'think aloud' until they reached a conclusion on how they perceived the particular issue (Legard, Keegan and Ward, 2003).

Following data collection, digital voice recordings were transcribed verbatim and subjected to a thematic analysis, based on the 'Framework' approach of Ritchie and Lewis (2003). This analytical approach reduced and organised the data into categories and overall themes, representing the participants' experience and perceptions of gender and speech and language therapy.

Findings

The male perspective

Convenience sampling led to a sample of three male student speech and language therapists and two female speech and language therapists. Themes identified in the participants' responses reflected those existing in the wider and profession-specific literature, including: *awareness of the profession, salary and promotion, male/female divide, working with children* and *perceived gender roles*.

Awareness

Participants were either directly aware of speech and language therapy as a career or had become interested in it by chance. For example, one participant reported that he found the work "she" did interesting and said that it influenced his decision to follow a similar career

> I had speech therapy when I was like ten or something... but I didn't really think of it as a career until [college]... If I didn't have a stammer I don't think I would have known speech therapy was an actual profession. Obviously it's, like, quite mainstream in health care, but it's still quite low key.

> I didn't know what I wanted to do and I just saw it on like a ... I did this, like, NHS test... you put in, like, some skills and it said, like, what careers would suit you and speech therapy was one of the top ones.

Experiences as a student

Participants were not expecting the number of females there were on their courses upon joining.

> I was aware that the industry was quite female dominated but I really wasn't expecting to be the *only* male on the course... that was a bit of a surprise... I was aware that there would be a gender bias but I had no idea it was quite this bad.

> I was expecting that there might be, like, a few more guys, like, when I first turned up, that was a bit of a shock on the first day.

However neither were noticeably affected by this.

> I've worked in a female dominated environment before so when I was surrounded by females on the course I wasn't too fazed because I'm used to it.

Salary and promotion

The males in this study expressed a neutral consideration to the remuneration of a speech and language therapist. Neither student had factored salary into their decision to study on the course. One participant was more concerned about being promoted but perhaps not for the reasons of attaining more responsibilities and receiving a higher salary. Another participant, although not preoccupied by career progression, thought this was an important consideration for males in general.

> [Salary and promotion] didn't figure in my choice of being a speech and language therapist, at all. I was pleasantly surprised when another student on the course told me how much a speech and language therapist could earn. I knew it was more than I was currently paid being a communication support assistant... I would assume that men are more interested in going for promotions. Personally I wanted to do a job to work with kids, but I wouldn't be adverse to it.

> I don't really know what the management for speech therapy is so I would say I like the practical side of it, definitely to start off with anyway, then, like, after a bit you can see, if you don't enjoy it, you can go to the management... You don't really want to stay on the same stage... I think that's a general thing. I think you'd get bored if you stay at the same level.

Male/female divide

Discussions about the advantages of being male, within this female-dominated profession, emerged. One participant discussed the idea that there may be more opportunity for advancement in the career by being male. There were also converging ideas about males being 'better' role models for male clients in receipt of speech and language therapy.

> I think it's definitely an advantage, being a male in the speech and language profession... well, I don't know, I guess, I would assume that because, there are so many women, in the speech and language profession, I guess that if you're a bloke, you'll stand out won't you? So even without trying, you're going to be more obvious.

> Hopefully it'll be good when I go to get a job and stuff, because if there aren't many guys that do it then they might be, like, maybe, they will want to get a few more guys or whatever... but if you went to a job, the guy wouldn't, might not necessarily get it over women, it's still down to whoever's got the best assets.

Advantages of being male were also discussed with regards to the high number of male clients.

> I guess at the very least 50 percent of the client base will be male, so the boys will see men as role models and perhaps my managers will think, well, this person is male, and this client is male, so I may be given more case loads.

> Quite a lot of people with speech impediments are guys so…
> I might be able to like bond a little bit… hopefully it'll be
> nice to connect with, like, kids who are the same gender.

Isolation was a theme that emerged from both interviews with students. One said that when he worked in the secondary school prior to joining the course, he was with middle-aged, middle-class, white females who have "specific topics of conversation". He explained that he felt a bit left out of the conversation. However, one participant also suggested that he would only feel like this with certain members of the female staff and debated that it could have been due to personality and had they not have been female, they may still have excluded him from conversation. He found the same situation on the course and said he was "not automatically part of the natural, social clique".

Another participant felt the same.

> If they're talking about girls' stuff like clothes or whatever,
> it's just like… (*rolled eyes to show boredom*)… but I've spent
> a lot of time with my girlfriend so I'm used to that… it's
> all right.

From a client's point of view, one participant mentioned the differences between males and females.

> I preferred a female [speech and language therapist]. I feel
> more relaxed sometimes around women especially when
> you, it's a little bit more personal, and I prefer to talk to
> females… I think that's just because, when I stammer, I tend
> to stammer more in front of guys than I do women.

This participant actually surmised that, perhaps subconsciously, he perceived males as more aggressive which rendered him less at ease among males.

Working with children

One participant had worked within a group of two females whilst on the placement in the primary school. He reported that some of the support staff would respond more positively to him than they would to the females when asking questions about resources, i.e., asking for photocopies, and thought this was due to his gender. However, he went on to say that his age may have been a possible factor. Whilst on this placement, he also noticed that there were different rules for the females than for him.

> I was instructed to, when working with a student, on my own, in a room, to not leave the door shut, to let the child sit between me and the door and make sure there was another member of staff in the next room... I don't recall that conversation being held with any of my female colleagues.

He also expressed that he would be watched by members of the public.

> I have had some very odd looks from the public [when working with children] from women, actually, in the same area, looking at me as if I was someone to be wary of... I'd imagine in her mind she's thinking he probably has nothing to do with all these little kids but there's this man talking to all these little kids so I'll keep my eye on him.

One participant was unaware of the meaning of the word 'safeguarding' and was unable to discuss this topic as fully as Participant A. However, both participants expressed being at times uncomfortable with working with children in general. One participant talked in detail about the experiences he had had with children having worked in the secondary school. He talked about one specific day trip to a swimming pool.

> A young girl asked me... she was visually impaired and she needed help getting dressed, she asked me if her costume was on correctly. That's a valid question, a girl wouldn't want to go out into the pool with a badly adjusted swimsuit, so it was a reasonable request, I felt. So I said "It does appear OK to me, if you do have another question like that, please would you go and see someone else."

Another incident one participant spoke about was when a girl had fallen down a flight of steps and hurt herself.

> I took her to the nurse's room but the nurse wasn't present and I was well aware that any other female colleagues would

> have mopped up the blood from the knee, there's no way I would have done that... because an adult male touching the knee of a girl could have been perceived in a way that I'm uncomfortable with... my first aiding abilities were adequate for the task. I would have been less concerned [had she been a boy] but I would still have preferred a female around because they were a child.

Gender roles

During the interviews, each participant was asked their opinion on gender roles and how this impacts on their behaviours and attitudes towards speech and language therapy. Also, they were asked why they think fewer males enter into speech and language therapy than females.

> I think I'm quite an empathetic, sympathetic person, but I do understand that those are considered quite feminine traits... I don't think that's necessarily the case but I think, socially, men, aren't penalised, but it's kind of assumed that men aren't going to get too emotional or even just empathise with other people's feelings in situations. It's not necessarily something a man would automatically be expected to do but I have no truck with that.

Another participant commented:

> I don't know really if it's because guys are, like, masculine or, like, macho or whatever and, like, can't see themselves doing a caring role... maybe they're just, like, socialised to be like brick or something.

The female perspective

This sample included two female speech and language therapists, with experience of working with male speech and language therapists and supervision of male speech and language therapy students.

These participants were asked, "What is your overall perception of male speech and language therapists in the profession?"

One participant replied:

> Often I think the men in our profession are much, maybe better… than women at looking at the career strategically, if that make sense? Yeah, generally I never really perceived [that], in terms of clinical skills I think all the guys I have worked with have been consistently excellent.

Interestingly, the other participant focused on positive outcomes.

> I think it would be better for the profession, because I think it would improve things, like our structure, if we had more men.

Indeed, both participants mentioned that they believe males bring benefits to their profession. One participant, when talking about males, also said

> …I think they do add something different into the mix.

This implies that professional female speech and language therapists perceive that having more men in a predominantly female environment would be beneficial, firstly to the workplace environment itself, but furthermore to the ability to provide suitable care to patients; that the differing skills and perceptions of men would create better care.

One of the participants discussed their experience of mentoring a male student. Their student had reported that numerous professionals had behaved 'differently' towards him than with his female counterparts. The student was described as male, and approximately in his late 30s, early 40s.

> He felt that his practice educators were perhaps a little bit wary of him and maybe… not frightened but a little bit intimidated by him because… [of] his age and his gender…, so yes that's one recent incident I've had that… certainly a male student has felt that he was perceived differently because of his gender.

Another participant expressed the belief that the majority of men who do take a career in speech and language therapy are inclined to avoid practice and stay in a more high status role in lecturing or research:

> ... because I've been more involved in the research area, I have come across quite a few [men], but they have all been in... the academic area, so much more in lecturing and in teaching than out in practice.

"In your opinion, what would inspire males to become speech and language therapists?"

In response to this prompt, responses from the two female participants were conflicting. One participant believed that the inspirations for a man would be for similar reasons as a woman and explained that it would be to gain the 'privilege' of working alongside clients.

Another participant stated that she thought it would be for different reasons, for example, salary being a big influence. Her response was:

> I suspect more money although it's not too badly paid these days but yes more money.

Participants were also asked: *"What is your overall perception of male speech and language therapists in the profession?"*

One participant said that all of the male speech and language therapists she worked with were 'consistently excellent'. Interestingly, she also stated that she believes them to be more ambitious and more career-minded than female speech and language therapists.

> ...very career focused, often I think the men in our profession are much um maybe better than the women at looking at career strategically if that makes sense?

Follow-up probes to this theme provided conflicting responses. One participant argued that males are not treated differently in the profession and that she had not come across anything similar to this.

These interviews, from female speech and language therapists, contribute to our understanding of gender and speech and language therapy. In particular, both participants suggested that males in the profession tend to be more ambitious and 'career focused', one participant even suggested that money might be an influencing factor as to why men aspire to become speech and language therapists, which was seen as a different aspiration to potential female speech and language therapists.

Another theme, though, that is evident in the findings was that both of the participants agreed that they would like to see more men qualifying into the profession. In particular, one participant expressed that she would like to know why more men do not enrol in this career and what could be done to improve this.

Overall, this data, from both males and females within the profession or training to enter it, has parallels between the differing perspectives sampled and with existing discourse and literature within the field. It could be argued that conflicting societal values lie at the heart of the situation. Whilst our society aspires to a balance of genders, within all professions, the reality is distant from this vision. The argument is better established from a female point of view and careers in management and science. Yet society, and individuals within it, are more ambivalent towards males in traditionally female careers. Although within organisations there are visions and strategies to increase the number of males entering caring and educational roles, cultural values regarding masculinity and social attitudes to men and safeguarding confuse the situation. In short, although there is a desire to increase men in caring and educational roles, this seems to be underlined by a suspicion that they are unsuitable to do so or, unlike females, are motivated less by altruism and more by incompatible aspirations for career progression.

Conclusion

From the male perspective, the challenges presented by speech and language therapy seem to be the same for both students and registered practitioners. In particular, these relate to working with children and young people and engaging with the working culture. Speech and language therapy as a profession faces the challenge of diversifying its workforce in the future, which is something that needs to happen alongside cultural changes in beliefs about the gendered division of labour and attitudes to males working with children and young people. Although a discussion of these social changes is outside the scope of this chapter, it is possible from the review of the literature and primary data presented to make some recommendations.

In particular, we could look at the development of peer support for male students and therapists. Whilst training and practicing, although it is a challenge to work with other males, it could be beneficial to encourage mentorship with male students or co-workers from other professions with a similar gender demographic. Indeed, special interest groups help to form a community for minority groups within industries. To help support male speech and language therapists, Australian clinicians have formed a group called 'Blokes in Speech Pathology', which helps to give role models to trainee males and form friendships with other males within this female dominated profession (McKinson, 2007).

Male students and therapists could also be encouraged and supported to specifically reflect on the influence their gender has on their practice and workplace relationships and the strategies they share to manage the experience. Furthermore, supervising clinicians and registered colleagues may reflect on their own attitudes to males in the profession, particularly the potential for discriminatory practice around males and safeguarding. Ultimately, perhaps the following quote, from a male student therapist, captures the ideal sentiment:

> I'm not training to be a man or a woman, but a speech and language therapist. For me it doesn't matter whether you're a man or a woman, just that you have an interest in and a passion for understanding and helping people with communication needs.

References

Boyd, S. & Hewlett, N. (2001) The gender imbalance among speech and language therapists and students. *International Journal of Language and Communication Disorders*, 36, 167–172.

Breitenbach, E. (2006) Gender statistics: An evaluation. *EOC Working Paper Series*. 51, 1–143.

Byrne, N. (2007) Factors influencing the selection of speech pathology as a career: A qualitative analysis utilizing the systems theory framework. *Australian Journal of Career Development*, 16(7), 11–18.

Butler, J. (1990) *Gender Trouble, Feminism and the Subversion of Identity*. London: Routledge.

Cross, S. & Bagilhole, B. (2002) Girls' jobs for the boys? Men, masculinity and non-traditional occupations. *Gender, Work and Organization*, 9(2), 204–226.

Cushman, P. (2005) Let's hear it from the males: Issues facing male primary school teachers. *Teaching and Teacher Education*, 21, 227–240.

Cushman, P. (2010) 'You're not a teacher, you're a man': The need for a greater focus on gender studies in teacher education. *International Journal of Inclusive Education*, 16(8), 775–790.

Dahlborg-Lyckhage, E. & Pilhammar-Anderson, E. (2009) Predominant discourses in Swedish nursing. *Policy, Politics, & Nursing Practice*, 10(2), 163–171.

Equality and Human Rights Commission Triennial Review (2010). How fair is Britain? Equality, human rights and good relations in 2010, the first triennial review. *Equality and Human Rights Commission*. http://www.equalityhumanrights.com/sites/default/files/documents/triennial_review/how_fair_is_britain_-_complete_report.pdf

Fuller, P. (1996). Masculinity, emotion and sexual violence. In L. Morris & S. Lyon (Eds) *Gender Relations in Public and Private*. London: Macmillan Press.

Greenwood, N., Wright, J.A. & Bithell, C. (2006) Perceptions of speech and language therapy amongst UK school and college students: Implications for recruitment. *International Journal of Language and Communication Disorders*, 41(1), 83–94.

Holmes, M. (2007). *What is Gender? Sociological Approaches*. London: Sage.

Legard, R., Keegan, J. & Ward, K. (2003) In-depth interviews. In J. Ritchie & J. Lewis (Eds) *Qualitative Research Practice: A Guide for Social Science Students and Researchers*, pp.139–169. London: Sage.

Litosseliti, L. & Leadbeater, C. (2012) Speech and language therapy/pathology: Perspectives on a gendered profession. *International Journal of Language and Communication Disorders*, 48(1), 90–101.

Loan-Clarke, J., Arnold, J., Coombs, C., Bosley, S. & Martin, C. (2009) Why do speech and language therapists stay in, leave and (sometimes) return to the National Health Service (NHS)? *International Journal of Language and Communication Disorders*, 44(6), 883–900.

Lupton, B. (2000) Maintaining masculinity: Men who do 'women's work'. *British Journal of Management*, 11(special issue), S33–S48.

Meadus, R.J. & Twomey, J.C. (2011) Men student nurses: The nursing education experience. *Nursing Forum*, 46(4), 269–279.

McAllister, L. & Neve, B. (2005) Male students and practitioners in speech pathology: An Australian pilot study. In *Proceedings of the Speech Pathology Australia Conference*, 29 May–2 June 2005, Canberra A.C.T., pp.1–8.

McKinson, F. (2007) Why do men become SLTs. *RCSLT Bulletin*, April. Issue 660, 12–14.

Miers, M. (2000) *Gender Issues and Nursing Practice*. Basingstoke: Palgrave Macmillan.

Ministry of Justice. (2010) Conviction histories of offenders between the ages of 10 and 52 in England and Wales. *Statistics Bulletin*.

Norton, J. (2013) *What is speech and language therapy?* www.rcslt.org/speech_and_language_therapy/what_is_an_slt/

Oakley, A. (1972) *Sex, Gender and Society*. London: Temple Smith.

Office for National Statistics (ONS). (2013) Labour market statistics, January 2013. *Statistics Bulletin.*

Riddell, S. & Tett, L. (2006) *Gender and Teaching: Where Have All the Men Gone?* Edinburgh: Dunedin Academic Press.

Riddell, S. & Tett, L. (2010) Gender balance in teaching debate: Tensions between gender theory and equality policy. *International Journal of Inclusive Education,* 14(5), 463–477.

Ritchie, J. & Lewis, J. (2003) *Qualitative Research Practice. A Guide for Social Science Students and Researchers.* London: Sage.

Sex Discrimination Act (1975). London: HMSO.

Skelton, C. (2003). Male primary teachers and perceptions of masculinity. *Educational Review,* 55(2), 195–209.

The Office of the First Minister and Deputy First Minister (OFMDFM) (2011) Gender Equality Strategy Statistics: 2011 Update. www.OFMDFM.gov.uk.

Thornton, M. & Bricheno, P. (2000) Primary school teachers' careers in England and Wales: The relationship between gender, role, position and promotion aspirations. *Pedagogy, Culture and Society,* 8(2), 187–206.

Whittock, M. & Leonard, L. (2003) Stepping outside the stereotype. A pilot study of the motivations and experiences of males in the nursing profession. *Journal of Nursing Management,* 11(4), 242–249.

Wilson, E.M. (1998) Gendered career paths. *Personnel Review,* 27(5), 396–411.

Wright, J.A. & Kersner, M. (2009) *A Career in Speech and Language Therapy,* 2nd ed. London: Metacom Education.

Xu, Y. (2008) Men in nursing: Origin, career path, and benefits to nursing as a profession. *Home Health Care Management & Practice,* 21(1), 72–73.

9 A critical look at the concept of 'service' in speech and language therapy

Jane Stokes

This chapter explores the nature of the over-used word 'service'. Are we providing a service **for, with** or **to** people with communication disability? In the NHS are we public servants – whose needs are we serving? What is a Service User – and how does the word 'service' get used in describing our work?

Motivations of speech and language therapists

When interviewing prospective speech and language therapists, the most common reasons people give for wanting to be a speech and language therapist are that they want to make a difference, they want to help people, they want to be part of a profession that gives support to those with communication difficulties. An altruistic motivation to serve people, displaying a commitment to the public interest and compassion for others: these are the themes that come out of the discussion of their motivations. Whitehouse, Hird and Cocks (2007) investigated the reasons for the choice of speech and language therapy as a university subject. They found that three categories of responses emerged:

1. altruism
2. intellectual interest and
3. desire for a professional career.

This chapter explores the first of these – the desire for a career that responds to the altruism in speech and language therapy. Where does this desire come from? To what extent do we live up to our aspirations to be 'of service'? This topic is not widely explored in speech and language therapy literature and it may be useful for us to question our motivation. We think it is worth knowing how other professions have explored these topics. There are numerous relevant theories about motivation at work; one commonly used with people who go into the church, for example, is McLelland's human motivation theory (1961). This identifies three motivators: achievement, affiliation and power. As with other chapters in this book, by finding out how other professions have looked at this, we hope to shed light on the nature of the profession of speech and language therapy. By raising our awareness of our motivations, we can better protect ourselves from burnout, and be more conscious of the effect of our motivations on others with whom we work. By looking in more depth at the concept of 'service', we may gain insights into the nature of service user involvement, our relationship with service users and our effectiveness in achieving service user engagement.

In considering why we want to become speech and language therapists it is useful to consider the following. Does the desire to be a professional person who gains respect because of their knowledge and skills drive prospective speech and language therapists? Are speech and language therapists displaying public service motivation? Do we reflect sufficiently on the power imbalance inherent in the therapeutic relationships we engage in? Where does our desire to 'help' come from and can we benefit from more scrutiny of this desire? Do these motivations affect our ability to really collaborate with our service users?

Motives in those interested in becoming speech and language therapists have rarely been explored. An understanding of these motives can give support to students through their training and their professional lives. In raising our awareness of our motivations, we can provide a stronger foundation for attending to the clinical relationships that we develop with our clients, and develop our therapeutic use of ourselves as vehicles for change (Geller in Fourie, 2011). The limited research that exists into why people choose speech and language therapy frequently cites the desire to help others as featuring very strongly in people's motivations (Byrne, 2007; Lass et al., 1992–1993; Rockwood and Madison, 1992–1993; Stewart, Pool and Winn, 2002). In Byrne's study (2007), all respondents made reference to a personal desire to help others as a significant factor in their career selection. Responses such as "I get lots of pleasure from helping people and I just thought that I'd only be truly happy if I did something along those lines" were typical, along with an interest in the topic areas associated with speech and language therapy.

Becoming a professional person and public sector motivation

People may be drawn to becoming a speech and language therapist because it confers a professional label. Being part of a professional group entails a sense of respect from others. Being a professional person privileges knowledge vested in the profession. Professions are generally thought to be working for the common good, to have a professional organisation that monitors education and sets standards, professional group (Brante, 2010). These aspects may affect the choice of career.

The majority of speech and language therapists in the UK work in the public sector. As such, they are probably influenced by a motivation to serve the public. Perry and Wise (1990) defined public service motivation (PSM) as an individual's predisposition to respond to motives grounded in public institutions. Perry (1996) identified four dimensions: attraction to public policy making; commitment to the public interest and civic duty; compassion; and self-sacrifice. According to Perry (2000), PSM is developed through individual experiences including life events, socialisation from family influences and education and professional training. The primary factors influencing people's motivation to engage in public service arise from parental relations, religion, observational learning and modeling. Perry (1997) found that having a religious worldview had no significant impact. The extent to which people in public service had learned altruistic or helping behaviour from their parents had a strong positive effect. Whether or not people had a strong relationship with one or both parents had no impact. It is not known whether these factors influence people's choice of career as a speech and language therapist but certainly the desire to serve others is strongly represented in interviews of prospective speech and language therapists. In a review of the interview transcripts of prospective students on the Postgraduate Diploma in Speech and Language Therapy programme at the Universities of Medway, altruism, the desire to help others, is a strong motivator in these, occurring in over 85% of answers given to the question, "Why do you want to train as a speech and language therapist?" This may well influence therapists' motivation for their choice of career. With the increase in private and independent working in the UK, it would be interesting to reflect on whether the motivation for public service is maintained despite the need to work in a more corporate culture. What is the effect of the economic incentive? Andersen (2009) explored the motivations of public sector and private sector health professionals in Denmark and found that both groups have high public sector motivation, a motivation to serve the interests of a community.

Altruism

The topic of altruism has been relatively ignored in speech and language therapy professional literature. Wakefield (1993) looked at whether altruism is part of human nature and questioned whether there might be a tension between being professional and being altruistic. In looking at the motivations of people who become social workers, Stevens et al. (2012) consider the possibility that the choice of a career in social work combines the need in people to have a meaningful career with a desire to contribute to society's wellbeing, thus bringing together career and altruistic motives. They say that motivation is a "complex mixture of personal, idealistic, and professional intentions" (p.19) and through reflection at the start of their career students can be guided to consider how this relates to them. Orbach in Bondi et al. (2011) says:

> … our altruistic impulses…are linked to, in some cases, a personal need to be given to and/or recognized. This does not render our efforts meaningless, but it does mean that it is worth understanding the underbelly, and thus the complexity of our own impulses to give (p.150).

The impact of personal experience

It is certainly the case that people applying to become speech and language therapists often do so because they have had personal experience of speech and language therapy and feel that they would like to share this experience by becoming trained in the skills and knowledge themselves (Byrne, 2007). These experiences figure highly in the personal statements on the application forms on our programme. Some are strongly motivated to provide a service that is better than the one they have experienced, and others have been so impressed by what they have seen that they are inspired to emulate it. Online blogs talk about the fact that people want to give back, to help people, with one person saying of this "I get off on it!", and saying that seeing progress is rewarding. There is an implicit satisfaction in seeing progress that can be attributed to the therapist's input, yet this satisfaction may be misplaced, as it may or may not be due to the therapist's intervention that progress has occurred (http://www.reddit.com/r/slp/comments/1dxf0h/what_was_your_inspiration_to_study_slp_why_did/).

In exploring the lived experience of becoming an occupational therapist, Tryssenaar (1999) looks at the meaning of therapy and the vocational aspect of the profession. She refers to the three meanings of therapy: "to render 'divine service', to 'heal' and to 'garden'" (p.107). She also includes in the definition of the profession a willingness to serve and to minister to others. The vocational aspect of being an occupational therapist refers to the inner drive to perform a service, as having a calling. It is certainly likely that some aspects of these motivations play a part in the decision to become a speech and language therapist.

The motivation to help

It is recognised that there is the possibility that people are drawn to the helping professions because they have a strong need to be needed. They seek to fulfill this need by creating dependent relationships (Luterman in Fourie, 2011). Being needed can lead to increased self-esteem and a feeling of self-worth. In becoming a speech and language therapist, students should be encouraged to consider why they want to be a helper. Egan's seminal text *The Skilled Helper* (2013) usefully explores the nature of the helping relationship and helps student speech and language therapists examine their own desire to help. This is key to how students should be prepared for clinical practice. Hawkins and Shohet (2000) refer to the wish to care, to cure and to heal which may derive from a hidden need for power, with people surrounding themselves with people worse off and being able to direct parts of the lives of the people who need help (p.11). They also discuss the need to be liked, valued and to be seen to be doing one's best. They write perceptively on the possibility that people are in the caring professions because they have an "addiction to giving" (p.17), which may be a defence against being a person who themselves needs support. Downs in Fourie (2011) talks about the fact that helping can sometimes verge on rescuing and that this can lead to dependency in the therapist's relationships. This dependency may not be something that the therapist is aware of. We do not believe that it has been much discussed in speech and language therapy. Useful discussion could emerge through skilled supervision, which could support the therapist in increasing their self-awareness. The bigger picture of exploring why we want to be helpers would benefit from wider discussion in the profession.

It is always possible that people resist being given help. By offering help, the implication is that people who are helped must accept it (Payne, 2011). This presents a challenge to the speech and language therapist when the client perhaps fails to attend. The acceptance that they need help is not always easy for someone and acutely disempowering for the client. Payne (2011) also points to the contradiction between the act of caring, which is construed as a personal response to someone else's condition and the professional responsibility for caring to have an evidence base drawn from science. We must beware of assuming that caring or helping is so self-evidently right that we do not think critically about it. By its very nature, helping is an 'outsider activity' (Payne, p.137) creating a distance between the helper and the helped.

Frank (2013) explores the concept of the wounded storyteller, and talks about the narratives that people tell about themselves in relation to illness (see also Chapter 6 for more discussion of this). Ferguson (2009) discusses the fact that these narratives do not construct the professional as a hero nor are patients expected to rise reborn, phoenix-like. Although this is perhaps an exaggerated view of how therapists may view themselves, much in Frank's writing can act as a corrective to the construing of therapy as helping.

There is benefit, too, in considering the relevance of the Jungian concept of the wounded healer. This relates to the phenomenon that many people in the helping professions have chosen that work because they themselves are 'wounded'. This can be a source of empathy and connectedness but is potentially detrimental to those in the position of being 'helped'.

Orbach in Bondi et al. (2011) talks about the personal motivations for doing the work we choose to do. In relation to psychotherapy, she considers that "the very reasons we are drawn to treat others may be out of some distress of our own, and we may be unconsciously hoping to solve, foist or resolve our own issues through a form of narcissistic gratification – giving to others what we long for ourselves" (p.145). She emphasises the importance of emotional self-knowledge as being protective to both our clients and to ourselves. Through skilled supervision by trained psychologists, speech and language therapists could be supported to explore these issues but, in practice, supervision is usually offered not by psychologists but by more senior speech and language therapists (see Chapter 3) who may not have the skills to engage in fuller discussion of such issues.

Issues of power

O'Malley (in Fourie, 2011) has explored issues of power in clinical discourse. She examines the asymmetry in the relationship between speech and language therapist and client. She suggests that being a client involves being in a relatively powerless position in terms of topic choice, maintenance, meaning and termination. She points to the usefulness of discourse analysis in exploring these unequal relationships. Ferguson and Armstrong (2004) examine the relationships between the professional expert (the speech and language therapist) and the client and consider the powerlessness that may ensue from this. Pillay (2003) refers to the dependency roles that clients are placed in and to the mismatch between the powerful expert and the sick person (in Kronenberg et al., 2011). Pound (2011) explores reciprocity and the supportive relationships between people with aphasia experienced at the UK charity for people with aphasia, Connect (www.ukconnect.org). The interactions of support they engage in are "uncluttered by the hierarchical power relationships inherent in therapy sessions and groups" (p.197). She quotes Oliver (2003) as saying that "rehabilitation is the exercise of power by one group over another" (p.38).

There are arguments that professions can contribute to an institutionalised form of client control. Illich et al. (1977) argued that professions are disabling, taking away the ability of people to decide for themselves. Others (Freidson, 1960) have drawn attention to the tendency of professions to monopolise knowledge. Hammell (2011) talks of theoretical imperialism in occupational therapy and Pillay in Kronenberg et al. (2011) draws parallels between colonialism and the helping professions in the ethnocentricity of their approach. These arguments all relate to the power imbalances that characterise the relationship between speech and language therapist and client or service user.

Because the therapist can communicate and he or she is working with someone who cannot communicate there is a very delicate balancing act to be made between advocating for someone, and speaking for them. Togher, Hand and Code (1996) draw attention to the disempowerment that results from children or adults not having equal access to the power of language.

Facilitated communication, a technique where the therapist provides a degree of physical support to a client in order to assist their communication, is a highly controversial approach and clearly calls into question the authorship of any message communicated by this technique. It is infrequently used with people with autism in the UK and there are conflicting views amongst practitioners about its efficacy. More routinely, speech and language therapists are often asked for their specialist advice for example on approaches to working with autism and have to use their professionalism in ensuring that they do not make decisions for people but with them. Some members of the autism community question approaches which work towards normalisation, but as a profession speech and language therapy has not really worked out a response to this, leaving the individual speech and language therapist managing the power challenges this can present. The work that has developed recently with young offenders also calls into question issues of power, with speech and language therapists working with disenfranchised people in subcultures quite removed from their own personal and professional cultures.

People with communication disorders are often seen as having a problem and experts as having the solutions. That is the way that the health service is set up; you are referred, you are seen, intervention is carried out, you are treated. Practitioners are accountable to the system that they work in, they have to account for their time, comply with the system requirements. Ferguson (2009) talks about speech and language therapists as "agents of the social structure that gives rise to a profession that attempts to bring individuals towards the predominant pattern" (p.105). People with communication disabilities enter into a therapeutic relationship with their speech and language therapist from a position of vulnerability (Sherratt and Hersh, 2010). There is an inherent power differential.

Ferguson (2009) used critical discourse analysis to shed light on the power relations in the culture of speech and language therapy by examining the language used in three statements about the profession's scope of practice, from USA, Canada and Australia.

> Terms reflecting an imbalance of power toward the speech language pathologist (e.g., select, prescribe, discharge, instruct, administer, train, supervise) were used more often than less powerful terms (e.g., service, serve). It was notable that terms around the concept of collaboration (e.g., refer, consult, collaborate, negotiate) only occurred in relation to other professionals and not in relation to clients… (p.108).

Ferguson (2009) comments that people with communication and swallowing disorders "… are strikingly absent from these documents at numerous levels… the discourse placed the client as passive recipient of the services" and comments on "the complexity in our role, both when working as agents of our own institutions, as well as on a day to day basis when working with clients" (p.110).

Ferguson (2009) also draws attention to the paradox involved in trying to 'treat' and at the same time 'facilitate adjustment' (p. 110). As Ferguson says elsewhere (2008) so many of the theories that inform an understanding of communication disorders are deficit-oriented. This characterises the relationships that we develop with our service users.

Horton (2006) discusses how therapists attempt to give explanations to the clients but it is hard for them to understand the reasoning behind the tasks. As Ferguson (2009) points out, without being able to negotiate toward a shared understanding of the point of therapy, then the goals of clients in therapy may never be met (Worrall et al., 2006). By using words like 'good' in response to a client's utterance, the implication is that the expert is judging the communication (Ferguson, 2009, p.110).

Power relations within service user involvement

Service user involvement is now built into the fabric of the helping professions. Service user participation underpins the work of the NHS. In a document published by NHS England, *Everyone Counts; Planning for Patients 2014/15 to 2018/9*, citizen inclusion and empowerment are two of the key strands. But the challenge for us is in relinquishing the power vested in us as professional experts, and in revising our clinician-directed working practices.

Much of the user involvement is initiated and led by professionals. The routine of carrying out patient satisfaction surveys is generally something led by the priorities of the service, rather than deriving from the experience of the client.

Fudge, Wolfe and McKevitt (2008) found little evidence that user involvement directly contributed to improved quality of services except in a few limited areas. This is largely because there is no agreed measure of success against which to compare service user involvement. So often we do not involve users of the service in strategic planning, generating ideas, or training of staff. These are missed opportunities. The influence of service users may be limited because they are often consulted on plans, priorities and goals that have already been devised rather than being involved in drawing these up in the first place.

Looking at issues of our professional motivation, desire to help and power relationships can add depth to our understanding of what true service user involvement demands of us. In the profession we have mostly looked at the mechanics of service user involvement, the structures and systems that can be set up to support it. There has been discussion of the ladder of participation, and much discussion of collaborative goal setting, but it is just as important for us to reflect on the roots and influences on our personal motivations to gain an insight into this area. We need to pay attention to our personal and collective values to support us in maintaining our professional motivations. Byng, Cairns and Duchan (2002) importantly raise this point, drawing attention to the risks of burnout or disillusionment if we do not focus on our values. They report on therapists who went into the job because they wanted to help others but who find that prevailing cultures and systems make it hard for them to practise in a way that is consistent with their values. Ross in Fourie (2011) discusses the links between unresolved issues such as "the need to be needed… the need to rescue people …which tend to disempower and foster dependent relationships among clients" (p.219).

If we do not pay attention to our values, and fail to remind ourselves of our motivations, we risk putting barriers in the way of real service user empowerment by persisting in relationships of dependency, where decisions are made **for** our clients instead of **with** them. Simmons-Mackie and Damico (2011) look in detail at the behaviour of therapists who control turns, take the lead on evaluating performance, request information that is already known, thereby reinforcing the powerless nature of the client in receipt of therapy. This can potentially reduce the ability of the service user to be able to contribute to either individual care planning or larger service planning issues. This behaviour, arising from unconscious and unexplored issues in the therapist's attitudes and beliefs, may actively impede service user involvement. To shift the emphasis from relationships that perpetuate the patient as passive recipient may require a large-scale culture change within the profession that has not yet been fully acknowledged.

There are examples of some excellent projects involving service users which shine out as leading the field in speech and language therapy. The Palin Parent Rating Scale (Fall 2013 Stuttering Foundation Newsletter) is an example of a tool that was developed in collaboration with parents. Galliers et al. (2012) looked at designing a therapy tool in collaboration with people with aphasia which again serves as a great example of true participation of people with aphasia in the research process. They talk about the shift that takes place for the speech and language therapists when collaborating in the research project; a shift from viewing the collaborator as patient to colleague.

This challenged some of the participant speech and language therapists' preconceptions of themselves as 'fixers'. The concept of the expert patient has been gaining ground recently but has yet to establish itself in the literature of speech and language therapy.

The predominant discourse that student practitioners are introduced to in their pre-registration education and placement experience is one based on the medical model; case history taking, session planning carried out by the therapist, decisions on prioritisation, discharge and directions to colleagues and family members. There is little or no discussion of disability studies or disability activism in relation to speech and language therapy and these topics do not constitute an essential part of the speech and language therapy curriculum. The Royal College of Speech and Language Therapists has only recently started to explore its role in supporting active service user participation in their policy and campaigning work. The Health and Care Professionals Council (HCPC), our regulatory body, has recently consulted with service users about changes to their standards of conduct, performance and ethics. This is ground-breaking work for the organisation and paves the way for further such work in future.

The term 'service user' has been explored by a group of service users involved in writing a document for the Social Care Institute for Excellence (SCIE, 2007). When asked to define the term 'service user', they identified the way in which the term may be used. They say:

> The term 'service user' can be used to restrict your identity as if all you are is a passive recipient of health and welfare services. That is to say, that a service user can be seen to be someone who has things 'done to them' or who quietly accepts and receives a service. This makes it seem that the most important thing about you is that you use or have used services. It ignores all the other things you do and that make up who you are as a person. (p.viii)

In work for the HCPC looking at the term 'service user' (2013), people who have used the service of allied health practitioners talked about how they construed the word. They emphasised the importance of service users as a term being based on self-identification:

> It means that we are in an unequal and oppressive relationship with the State and society.

> It is about entitlement to receive welfare services. This includes the past when we might have received them and the present.
>
> It may mean having to use services for a long time which separate us from other people and which makes people think we are inferior and that there is something wrong with us. (p.7)

Other terms have been tried out in place of 'service user', as the word 'user' is thought by some to have a passive connotation. Users are not grateful recipients of a service, but might best be seen as a consumer of a service. This in turn does not really reflect the reality of healthcare in the UK, as it implies that someone can choose from a range of services (Barnes and Cotterell, 2012). The term 'partner' has recently been widely used and implies a more equal relationship – which is often more an aspiration than a reality given the organisational structures that health practitioners traditionally work in.

These debates challenge the practitioner to continually ensure that they are viewing the person they are working with as not a passive recipient. But so many of our systems and processes are set up with a framework of asymmetrical relationships that it takes constant work on the part of the therapist to counter it. Power sharing can be difficult within established mainstream structures, formal consultation mechanisms and traditional ideologies (SCIE, 2007, p.13).

Swinburn in Anderson and van der Gaag (2005) feels that user involvement is more rhetoric than reality. As she says, true user involvement requires "time, commitment, courage and reflection" and "user involvement without culture change can be unproductive" (p.116). This culture change has not been wholesale within the field of speech and language therapy despite some important work in eliciting the views of people with communication difficulties (Merrick and Roulstone (2011), the Bercow Report (DCSF 2008) and projects described in the useful set of commissioning tools for speech, language and communication needs developed by the Communication Trust. The Francis Report (2013) placed the testimonies of patients in a central role in and the Keogh review (2013) used focus groups to gather information very effectively. Robson, Begum and Locke (2003) distinguish between two types of user involvement: management-centred user involvement where service users participate in existing structures but the organisations determine the content and the direction of this participation, and user-centred user involvement where the objectives of service users become the focus and priority of the organisation. There is evidence that when people with communication disorders are involved in participative approaches to planning services they experience benefits in confidence and feelings of self worth, which in turn has a rehabilitative effect (Burgess and Stansfield, 2010).

We need to make the shift from listening and consulting to collaboration and responsiveness and, embedded as we still are in a largely medical framework of thinking, there is plenty of work to do. We are encouraged to involve clients in the process of goal setting and outcome measurement but in reality goals and outcomes are often determined by the outcome of formal assessments rather than from real joint work with the clients. Clewley and Roberts (2014) describe a client-led service for people with aphasia, which allowed them to select an awareness raising project in which they wanted to be involved. We still have to develop this approach and incorporate it into how students are prepared for clinical work. Terms such as 'partnership' or 'co-creation', prevalent in the field of higher education, are not so widespread in the field of speech and language therapy and these concepts could certainly be usefully applied. Co-production, a practice described in the NHS Confederation document *Changing Care, Improving Quality* (2013) refers to the process whereby patients' organisations are involved in critiquing current provision and redesigning it to meet their needs and priorities. Concepts of co-design and co-production have much to teach us. These are collaborative relationships where service users and professionals share power and have equal ability to contribute to service developments.

Experience based co-design is another approach which has been given more emphasis recently but we have a long way to go in speech and language therapy to embed this in our research (http://www.kingsfund.org.uk/projects/ebcd).

Services are continually being reconfigured in speech and language therapy but rarely put the clients at the centre of this process. Law et al. (2010) discuss the challenges involved in the recognition that the views of people with aphasia about services do not always coincide with those of service providers. Connect, the UK-based charity, has a central and very strong ethos of placing the user at the centre of the service, and has led the way in the profession on this approach. We need to continue to learn from our colleagues in other parts of the health service and primarily from service user organisations about this approach.

Anderson and van der Gaag (2005) contrast the "profession-led perspective where the professional sees herself as expert on a condition versus the client-led perspective where the client is the expert" (p.3). The profession of speech and language therapy still casts itself more in the first mould.

The concept of service, of caring, and the activities of therapy

The term 'being of service to someone', as implied in the phrase 'service provider' has connotations of doing something to someone, doing them a favour, doing them a kindness, or being of assistance. However, we must be aware of the effect of this relationship on the people we work with. Kronenberg et al. (2005) argued that occupational therapists must "think and act critically, become aware of the value patterns and assumptions embedded in our theories and avoid contributing to the oppression of the very people we intend to help" (p.xvi).

In the speech and language therapy profession there is a strong humanistic focus but one that is not perhaps routinely made explicit. In line with humanistic social work there is an aspiration to practise in ways that facilitate the clients' experience of using their own knowledge and skills. There is a professional imperative that we should maintain a focus on personal growth and development for clients. But there is much about speech and language therapy that is prescriptive and counter to this model of working. The concept of a therapeutic alliance is a useful one, drawn from humanistic psychotherapy but, again, rarely discussed in speech and language therapy literature.

Simmons-Mackie and Damico in Fourie (2011) talk about therapy as not a unidirectional process of clinician 'doing to' a client but a collaborative activity in which both parties work to effect change (p.36). This begins to alter the concept of service to others. Luterman in Fourie (2011) talks about how we need to learn to be responsible **to** our clients, rather than being responsible **for** them. This is a fundamental shift in responsibility and calls into question concepts of care, service, helping. Care as a concept has been viewed by disability activists as oppressive and objectifying (Fine and Glendinning, 2005) yet little has been written about the dangers of this in speech and language therapy.

Kovarsky (2008) says that current models of evidence-based practice marginalise and even silence the voices of those who are the potential beneficiaries of assessment and therapy. Lewis (2001) succinctly captures the role of evidence in the knowledge base for social care in the formula:

> Knowledge = evidence + practice wisdom and service user and carer experiences and wishes

This combination of factors which she sees as making up professional knowledge could certainly apply to speech and language therapy. The issue for us is a potential weighting of evidence over service user and carer experiences and a possibility that we minimise the importance of the latter over the former. We must find ways of raising the importance of service user experience as a form of evidence and seeing it as key to the provision of effective therapy.

Simmons-Mackie and Damico (1999) refer to the interactional asymmetry in traditional impairment-focused therapy. It may be more helpful to look, as Mattingly does in relation to occupational therapy (1998), at the idea of therapeutic plots – secular rituals that help patients make the transition from illness reality to new reality and even a new self. She places value on improvisation in therapy, a process which allows for more equal participation by both partners in the relationship.

Conclusion

This chapter has aimed to briefly explore the concepts of service and serving and how these relate to speech and language therapy. The intention is to stimulate reflection on this important topic. In conclusion, the reader is referred to the work of Rachel Naomi Remen, Clinical Professor of Family and Community Medicine at the University of California in San Francisco and a pioneer in the holistic health movement. Remen (1996) explores the connected processes of helping, fixing and serving, which she sees as representing three different ways of seeing life. She privileges the concept of serving over helping and fixing and her work is a call to rethink the concept of service.

> When you help, you see life as weak. When you fix, you see life as weak. When you serve, you see life as whole. Fixing and helping may be the work of the ego, and service the work of the soul.
>
> Seeing yourself as a fixer may cause you to see brokenness everywhere, to sit in judgment of life itself. When we fix others, we may not see their hidden wholeness or trust the integrity of the life in them. Fixers trust their own expertise. When we serve, we see the unborn wholeness in others;

we collaborate with it and strengthen it. Others may then be able to see their wholeness for themselves for the first time. (Remen, 1996, p.25)

This is a more positive slant on the term 'to serve', free of the complexities of one's own possible unacknowledged motivations. What is clear is, that as Luterman in Fourie (2011) says, being in service to the other is very demanding. The most important clinical tool is still the clinician. So it is the clinician that needs to continually examine and scrutinise his or her motivations, values, and belief systems to ensure that they continue to do something **with** the client rather than **to** the client. This should be a constant theme in reflective practice and supervision when working as a speech and language therapist.

References

Andersen, L. (2009) What determines the behaviour and performance of health professionals? Public service motivation, professional norms and/or economic incentives. *International Review of Administrative Sciences*, 75(1), 79–97.

Anderson, C. & van der Gaag, A. (2005) *Speech and Language Therapy: Issues in Professional Practice*. Chichester: John Wiley & Sons.

Barnes, M. & Cotterell, P. (Eds) (2012) *Critical Perspectives on User Involvement*. Bristol: The Policy Press.

Bondi, L., Carr, D., Clark, C. & Clegg, C. (2011) *Towards Professional Wisdom: Practical Deliberation in the People Professions*. Farnham: Ashgate.

Brante, T. (2010) Professional fields and truth regimes: In search of alternative approaches. *Comparative Sociology*, 9, 843–886.

Department for Children, Schools and Families (2008) The Bercow Report: A Review of Service for Children and Young People (0–19) with Speech, Language and Communication Needs. http://webarchive.nationalarchives.gov.uk.

Burgess, R. & Stansfield, J. (2010) Lighting the touch paper: Empowering stroke patients through service user involvement. *International Journal of Stroke*, 5(S3), 45.

Byng, S., Cairns, D. & Duchan, J. (2002) Values in practice and practising values. *Journal of Communication Disorders*, 35(2), 89–106.

Byrne, N. (2007) Factors influencing the selection of speech pathology as a career: A qualitative analysis utilising the systems theory framework. *Australian Journal of Career Development*, 16(3), 11–17.

Clewley, K. & Roberts, J. (2014) Communicating with confidence. The voice newsletter. Royal College of Speech and Language Therapists: Wales. http://www.rcslt.org/governments/docs/voice_jan2014_english

The Communication Trust Speech and Language Commissioning Tools. https://www.thecommunicationtrust.org.uk/commissioners/slcn-commissioning-tools.aspx

Egan, G. (2014) *The Skilled Helper: A Problem Management and Opportunity-development Approach to Helping*, 10th ed. Brooks Cole. Belmont: Cengage Learning.

Ferguson, A. (2008) *Expert Practice: A Critical Discourse*. San Diego: Plural Publishing.

Ferguson, A. (2009) The discourse of speech-language pathology. *International Journal of Speech-Language Pathology*, 11, 104–112.

Ferguson, A. & Armstrong, E. (2004) Reflections on speech-language therapists' talk: Implications for clinical practice and education. *International Journal of Language and Communication Disorders*, 39, 469–477.

Fine, M. & Glendinning, C. (2005) Dependence, independence or inter-dependence? Revisiting the concepts of 'care' and 'dependency'. *Ageing and Society*, 25, 601–621.

Fourie, R. (2011) *Therapeutic Processes for Communication Disorders: A Guide for Clinicians and Students*. Hove: Psychology Press.

Francis, R. (2013) *Report of the Mid-Staffordshire NHS Foundation Trust Public Inquiry*. London: The Stationery Office. https://www.gov.uk/government/publications/report-of-the-mid-staffordshire-nhs-foundation-trust-public-inquiry.

Frank, A. (2013) *The Wounded Storyteller: Body, Illness and Ethics*, 2nd ed. Chicago: University of Chicago Press.

Freidson, E. (1960) Client control and medical practice. *American Journal of Sociology*, 65, 374–382.

Fudge, N., Wolfe, C. & McKevitt, C. (2008) Assessing the promise of user involvement in health service development: ethnographic study. *British Medical Journal*, 336, 313–317.

Galliers, J., Wilson, S., Roper, A., Cocks, N., Marshall, J., Muscroft, S. & Pring, T. (2012) Words are not enough: Empowering people with aphasia in the design process. In *Proceedings of the 12th Participatory Design Conference 1*, pp.51–60. New York: Association for Computing Machinery.

Hammell, K. (2011). Resisting theoretical imperialism in the disciplines of occupational science and occupational therapy. *British Journal of Occupational Therapy*, 74, 27–33.

Hawkins, P. & Shohet, R. (2000) *Supervision in the Helping Professions*, 2nd ed. Buckingham: Open University Press.

Health and Care Professionals Council (2013) *Shaping our Lives. Service User and Carer Consultation: Review of the Standards of Conduct, Performance and Ethics of the Health and Care Professions Council*. http://www.hcpc-uk.org/assets/documents/10004528HCPCreportbyShapingOurLivesfinal.pdf

Horton, S. (2006) A framework for description and analysis of therapy for language impairment in aphasia. *Aphasiology*, 20(6), 528–564.

Illich, I., Zola, I., McKnight, J., Caplan, J., & Shaiken, H. (1977) *Disabling Professions*. London: Marion Boyars.

Keogh B. (2013) *Review into the Quality of Care and Treatment Provided by 14 Hospital Trusts in England: An Overview Report*. www.nhs.uk/NHSEngland/bruce-keogh-review/Documents/outcomes/keogh-review-final-report.pdf

The King's Fund. Experience-based co-design toolkit. http://www.kingsfund.org.uk/projects/ebcd

Kovarsky, D. (2008) Representing voices from the life-world in evidence-based practice. *International Journal of Language and Communication Disorders*, 43, 47–57.

Kronenberg, F., Simó Algado, S. & Pollard, N. (Eds) (2011) *Occupational Therapy without Borders: Learning from the Spirit of Survivors*. London: Elsevier-Churchill Livingstone.

Lass, N., Middleton, G., Pannbacker, M. & Marks, C. (1992–1993) A survey of speech-language pathologists' career development and satisfaction. *National Student Speech Language Hearing Association Journal*, 20(1), 99–104.

Law, J., Huby, G., Irving, A.-M., Pringle, A.-M., Conochie, D., Haworth, C. & Burston, A. (2010) Reconciling the perspective of practitioner and service user: Findings from The Aphasia in Scotland study. *International Journal of Language & Communication Disorders*, 45(5), 551–560.

Lewis, J. (2001) What works in community care? *Journal of Integrated Care*, 9(1), 3–6.

Mattingly, C. (1998) *Healing Dramas and Clinical Plots: The Narrative Structure of Experience*. Cambridge: Cambridge University Press.

McLelland, D. (1961) *The Achieving Society*. Princeton NJ: Van Nostrand.

Merrick, R. & Roulstone, S. (2011) Children's views of communication and speech-language pathology. *International Journal of Speech-Language Pathology*, 13(4), 281–290.

Pillay, M. (2011) (Re-)habilitation and (re)positioning the powerful expert and the sick person. In: F. Kronenberg, N. Pollard & D. Sakellariou (Eds) *Occupational Therapies Without Borders. Volume 2: Towards an Ecology of Occupation-based Practices*. Edinburgh: Churchill/Elsevier.

NHS England (2013) *Everyone Counts; Planning for Patients 2014/15 to 2018/19*. http://www.england.nhs.uk/wp-content/uploads/2013/12/5yr-strat-plann-guid-wa.pdf

NHS Confederation (2013) *Changing Care, Improving Quality: Reframing the Debate on Reconfiguration*. http://www.nhsconfed.org/resources/2013/06/changing-care-improving-quality-reframing-the-debate-on-reconfiguration

Oliver, M. (2003?) *Understanding Disability: From Theory to Practice*. Basingstoke: Palgrave Macmillan.

The Palin Parent Rating Scale. Available at https://secure.psych.lse.ac.uk/Palin_Parent_Rating_Scales/pprs_connect.php

Payne, M. (2011) *Humanistic Social Work: Core Principles in Practice.* Basingstoke: Palgrave Macmillan.

Perry, J. (1996) Measuring public service motivation: An assessment of construct reliability and validity. *Journal of Public Administration Research and Theory*, 6(1), 5–22.

Perry, J. (1997) Antecedents of public service motivation. *Journal of Public Administration Research and Theory*, 7(2), 181–197.

Perry, J. (2000) Bringing society in: Toward a theory of public-service motivation. *Journal of Public Administration Research and Theory*, 10(2), 471–488.

Perry, J. & Wise, L. (1990) The motivational bases of public service. *Public Administration Review*, 50(3), 367–373.

Remen, R.N. (1996) In the service of life. *Noetic Sciences Review*, Spring.

Robson, P., Begum, N. & Locke, M. (2003) *Developing User Involvement: Working towards User-centred Practice in Voluntary Organisations.* Bristol: The Policy Press.

Rockwood, G. & Madison, C. (1992–1993) A survey of program section and expectations of current and prospective graduate students. *National Student Speech Language Hearing Association Journal*, 20, 88–98.

Social Care Institute for Excellence (2007) Developing Social Care: Service Users Driving Culture Change by Shaping our Lives. National Centre for Independent Living (www.scie.org.uk) and University of Leeds Centre for Disability Studies,

Sherratt, S. & Hersh, D. (2010) "You feel like family...". Professional boundaries and social model aphasia groups. *International Journal of Speech Language Pathology*, 12(2), 152–161.

Simmons-Mackie, N. & Damico, J.S. (1999) Social role negotiation in aphasia therapy: Competence, incompetence, and conflict. In: D. Kovarsky, J.F. Duchan & M. Maxwell (Eds) *Constructing (In)competence: Disabling Evaluations in Clinical and Social Interaction*, pp. 313–342. Mahwah, NJ: Erlbaum.

Simmons-Mackie N. & Damico J. (2011) Counseling and aphasia treatment: Missed opportunities. *Topics in Language Disorders*, 31(4), 336–351.

Stevens, M., Moriarty, J., Manthorpe, J., Hussein, S., Sharpe, E., Orme, J., Mcyntyre, G., Cavanagh, K., Green-Lister, P. & Crisp, B.R. (2012) Helping others or a rewarding career? Investigating student motivations to train as Social Workers in England. *Journal of Social Work*, 12(1), 16–36.

Stewart, S., Pool, J. & Winn, J. (2002). Factors in recruitment and employment of allied health students: Preliminary findings. *Journal of Allied Health*, 31(2), 111–116.

Togher, L., Hand, L. & Code, C. (1996) A new perspective in the relationship between communication impairment and disempowerment following head injury in information exchanges. *Disability and Rehabilitation*, 18(11), 559–566.

Tryssenaar, J. (1999) The lived experience of becoming an occupational therapist. *British Journal of Occupational Therapy*, 62(3), 107–111.

Wakefield, J.C. (1993). Philosophy of science and the evaluation of clinical theory: A reply to the Piepers. *Social Service Review*, 67, 654–666.

Whitehouse, A., Hird, K. & Cocks, N. (2007) The recruitment and retention of speech and language therapists: What do university students find important? *Journal of Allied Health*, 36(3), 131–136.

Worrall, L., Davidson, B., Hersh, D., Howe, T., Ferguson, A. & Sherratt, S. (2006) What people with aphasia want: Toward person-centred goal setting in aphasia rehabilitation. Research in progress. Unpublished manuscript, cited in A. Ferguson (2008) *Expert Practice: A Critical Discourse*. Abingdon: Plural Publishing.

10 In conclusion

Marian McCormick and Jane Stokes

"We make the road by walking."
(Horton and Freire, 1990)

The process of setting up a new pre-registration programme for speech and language therapists has afforded us huge opportunities to reflect on the profession. Although we have developed the curriculum in line with guidelines produced by the Royal College of Speech and Language Therapists (RCSLT), Health and Care Professionals Council (HCPC) and the Quality Assurance Agency (QAA), in devising it we have found that there are a number of ways to cut the cake. We have had the privileged role of observing, experimenting and reflecting on what makes a good speech and language therapist. We have listened to ourselves telling stories to the students, listened to the placement educators tell us what they value most about the profession, and where they have questions and concerns. This has made us look afresh at aspects of what we have done in our professional lives, and consider how to best prepare students for practice in a rapidly changing and demanding professional context. We have explored our professional and personal selves in relation to the students and considered and re-considered how best to present information, experience and knowledge. Our curiosity has been stimulated by countless incidents and conversations. We have been helped by so many people along the way. It has been a period of transformative learning for us. Through Nicki Weld's book on transformative supervision (2012), we have been introduced to the Maori concept of 'ako'. This describes a teaching and learning relationship where the educator is actively learning from the student. The teacher becomes the learner, and the learner the teacher. This concept acknowledges that new knowledge and understanding grows from shared learning experiences. The spirit of reciprocal learning has infused our programme from the start and has built an inclusive learning community, drawing on the experience and expertise of what the students bring to the programme and the contributions of the placement educators and visiting lecturers.

The contributors of these chapters are people with whom we have had some of these conversations, who have challenged us with ideas and constructive criticism to consider alternative viewpoints and to reflect on our decisions and choices. These collaborations have been vital in the development and strengthening of the programme. More importantly, though, the contributions are, in themselves, evidence of the principles of reflection, theoretically motivated enquiry, and scholarship in practice – each of the chapters has come directly out of the practice, interests and genuine curiosity of those who have written them.

The initial aims of this book were to:

- Raise some of the unexplored, received wisdom about the role of the speech and language therapist
- Add to the debates about the aims and objectives of the profession, by exploring some of the unspoken sets of values that often surround our work, and questioning what we do and why
- Examine some of the contexts for professional practice that are rarely explored
- Encourage colleagues and future therapists to challenge, question, and adapt, using critical appraisal skills combined with reflective practice.

Along the way these aims have changed and evolved, and gone beyond the specific and the categorical because, although each chapter was written independently, very clear themes emerged as the work came together, and the following ideas, concepts and constructs appeared time and again. This chapter draws together the tapestry of perspectives that have been presented and highlights some key points from each chapter which we hope will act as reflection points, discussion topics, and prompts to further exploration and action.

- **The nature of knowledge and the definition of competence.** We must acknowledge and explore the tensions between evidence-based practice and the intuitive, tacit aspects of professional practice. As Clark in Bondi et al. (2011) says, "evidence based practice is mute on the moral and political ends of the human service professions without an understanding of which they are ultimately meaningless" (p.59). Whilst not minimising the importance of continuing to establish a strong knowledge base, we must not ignore the importance of professional wisdom and accumulated knowledge. However, there is an imperative to scrutinise this received wisdom for partiality, prejudice and debatable practice. Hence the need to question our models of service delivery (Chapters 2 and 4) and lack of diversity (Chapters 7 and 8).

- **The development of professional identity and professional confidence.** Professional roles and professional identity need to be considered individually and collectively. It is vital to explore the process of 'becoming' a therapist through developing our self-awareness and self-management, which form the basis for values-based practice and education. We must pay attention to the process of becoming a therapist, not simply the product, and be mindful of our epistemological journey (Chapter 1). The importance of proving our worth and our effectiveness is central to developing our confidence as a profession. We must find a way of maintaining the improvisatory nature of speech and language therapy, the ability to respond to the twists and turns of a client's responses to intervention (Chapter 4) whilst keeping a close eye on recording outcomes, and following evidence-based care pathways (Chapter 2). This can be a challenge to our commitment to person-centred care.

- **The nature of the therapeutic relationship.** In examining clinical reasoning we must assign central importance to the therapeutic alliance. As a profession we should not minimise the importance of the therapeutic relationship. This is an area that we have perhaps not given enough credence to in speech and language therapy. In the search to ensure that our practice is evidence-based and scientific in its grounding, we have not been as confident as, for example, the profession of psychotherapy, in our assertions about the importance of the therapeutic relationship as being at the core of our work. There have been decades of scientific research examining this in psychotherapy (Norcross, 2011) yet in speech and language therapy we do not accord it the same importance, nor do we draw sufficiently on the research done in other professions about the therapeutic relationship. As Hinckley (2008) says: "the power of the clinician is more than a correctly completed assessment with a matching and well-implemented treatment plan. The power of the clinician is also who you are and who you are to the client" (p.xiv). Power relations in the helping professions have been explored elsewhere but have had limited exposure in speech and language therapy literature. We need to ensure that these issues are continually examined (Chapter 9), both individually and collectively, and be alive to the possibility that in working with people with limited voice we are inevitably in an unequal relationship. Simmons-Mackie and Damico (1999) talk about the inherent paradox of therapy where in designing therapy programmes we construct contexts where clients are more likely to perform incompetently so that errors can be fixed via repair work (Kovarsky, Kimbarow and Kastner, 1999). Rogers' work is influential here: "...the person-centred view drastically alters the therapist-patient relationship ... The therapist becomes the 'midwife' of change, not its originator. She places the final authority in the hands of the client ... The locus of evaluation, of decision, rests clearly in the client's hands" (Kirschenbaum and Henderson, 1990, p.382).

- **Professional narrative and enhancement**. Reflection must remain at the core of our professional lives (Chapter 1). We must understand that only by stepping back and looking at the profession from a distance can we grow and develop. We need to commit to continue to deepen our own personal self-awareness as well as engage in collective reflections of ourselves as a profession. As Kronenberg, Pollard and Sakellariou (2011) say of occupational therapy, "maybe we have been too preoccupied with what we do and how we do it, instead of connecting with who we are and how we operate both individually and collectively" (p.5).

- **The power of working and learning collaboratively within and across professional boundaries**. Speech and language therapy can learn much from other professions. We have seen in the chapters on reflective practice, supervision, service users, teaching and spirituality (Chapters 1, 3, 5, 6 and 9) that we share territory with social work, nursing, education and other health professions. We can benefit from the work done elsewhere on these topics and must remain open and alive to other ways of thinking, doing and becoming. We have plenty of growing still to do as a profession and only by learning from other more established professions will we be able to explore the full potential of our work. By examining other professional worlds we can better understand our own one, consider how we can improve our preparation of students and strengthen our professional identity.

Speech and language therapy as a profession has many sides to it, and draws on many different schools of thought. This is a source of its richness but also leads to uncertainties, and a lack of confidence about its identity. Uncertainties about our role can lead to hesitancy and inertia. We need to have the confidence to explore our own professional cultures. Professional practice throws us many challenges. The book has raised dilemmas and controversies and there may be things with which you agree or disagree. Some ideas you may feel comfortable with, others not so comfortable; some things may become clearer in the process of reading about them, others may lose clarity. There are points in every speech and language therapist's professional life where we think "Hmmm…"; we hope this book will do the same for you.

The process of exploring the profession has been an adventure. The more we study the world of speech and language therapy the more we realise its complex and multidimensional components. In thinking about how we prepare the students for professional life, we have tried to balance the importance of acquiring knowledge and skills with a focus on what Dall'Alba calls the process of becoming. "Learning to become a professional involves not only what we know and can do, but also who we are (becoming)" (2009, p.34).

Implications for practice

What has emerged from this venture is the clear idea that the development of professional identity, individually and collectively, is a process that is ongoing, dynamic and intimately linked with a collaborative ethos. One question that stands out for us as a conclusion from working on the book is how we as a profession might further develop that identity through working together to develop a way of acknowledging each individual's work; facilitating collaborative and reciprocal learning relationships; celebrating best practice and encouraging scholarship.

From our experiences in establishing and developing this programme for pre-registration speech and language therapists, we have come to appreciate the value, and see the impact, of working in a way which uses person-centred development as a strategy for professional development (Jasper, 2006), and which encourages and expects ownership of learning. These ideas of taking responsibility for and responding to the context of one's practice in an independent and accountable manner, are central to the definition of professionalism. Such an approach emphasises the need for each individual to develop self-awareness, self-management and self-assessment, all of which are key to the development of autonomous and effective practice, and to advancing clinical knowledge, skills and understanding.

To this end, we have developed within the programme an approach to the representation of reflective practice which draws on the constructs of professional narrative. It supports each individual in representing the personal development that has occurred for them over a specific period of time; the change in their understanding of and engagement with reflective practice, and the outcomes of that widened perspective. The approach draws on the principles of the MOSAIC model (Clarke and Moss, 2001), and critical pedagogy, which both have as central constructs an ethics of participation, an emphasis on transformative learning, and highlight the centrality of 'meaning-making' to effective learning and effective change.

The primary aim of our approach is to encourage students to take an ipsative approach to their professional development; that is, to identify and describe their own 'starting point' in terms of reflective practice and use this as a baseline from which they can narrate and assess their own progress in terms that are meaningful to them. Students are asked to generate, select, and prioritise activities and interactions that had a significant impact on their learning; to place those events into a narrative and describe the impact of that learning on their future practice. This allows them to develop a strong sense of their personal progress, to articulate their growing competence in the use of their understanding and skills, and to begin the process of construction of professional identity.

Extract from student work:

> Initially I struggled with the concept of no title for this essay. Looking for externally imposed rules, and structure to help me construct my argument I was essentially searching for the safety of the banking concept (Freire, 2002) teaching style. Nevertheless, as part of the process

of reflective writing, I have slowly come to understand there could be no given title just as there was never a right answer to find. A title would necessarily have been prescriptive, and imposed expectations: a pedagogical approach to a necessarily ipsative metacognitive process (McGuinness, 2005). I have finally learnt a most important lesson to take from this module: I need the courage to design my own way forward and take control of my learning journey."

When approached in this way, reflective practice places the individual in a research mode of thinking, and touches on the principles of Grounded Theory (GT) (Glaser and Strauss, 2012). A major component of Grounded Theory research is the method of comparative analysis, which involves an ongoing process of data collection and analysis, leading to constant comparison between sets of information. "As issues of interest are noted in the data, they are compared with other examples for similarities and differences. Through the process of constant comparison … emerging theoretical constructs are continually being refined through comparisons with "fresh" examples from ongoing data collection, which produces the richness that is typical of grounded theory analysis... constant comparative analysis allows the integration of new and existing data in this iterative cycle, towards a well-grounded theory" (Lingard, 2008).

There are clear and important parallels between this research approach and critical reflective practice which, when approached in this manner, is intimately concerned with and linked to epistemological issues, specifically the growth and construction of professional knowledge.

The HCPC Standards of Education and Training (SETs), and Standards of Proficiency (SOPs), lay out a comprehensive and clearly-defined set of competencies for how we are expected to work, in line with its regulatory remit. They do not, however, aim to provide a framework for personal professional development. Such a framework would provide a means by which each therapist could represent the multiple dimensions of their practice, and link that practice, learning, skill development and knowledge to a professional progression pathway for post-qualifying education and training, which lays out aspirational stages of career development beyond registration.

The UK Professional Standards Framework (UKPSF) is an example of such a framework within the Higher Education sector. The appeal of such an approach is that it aims to provide a structure which arises from the sector – that is practitioner-led – and aims to recognise excellence, develop leadership, and provide a means for professional recognition and a framework for professional enhancement. It supports and encourages practitioners to describe how their continuing professional development (CPD) activities and clinical practice relate to their professional identity and progression.

Developing new areas of expertise, extending our roles or spheres of professional influence can be intimidating, but support and encouragement from within an inclusive and reciprocal learning environment can foster confidence and give us feedback as to the resources and skills others perceive in us. "True professionals have a full and bilateral relationship with knowledge: they do not only apply knowledge to their practice, but they also generate and disseminate it; that is they are researchers and educationalists as well as practitioners" (Rolfe, Jasper and Freshwater, 2010, p.31).

On the basis of our experiences, we propose an alternative or additional way of representing professional development and engagement within speech and language therapy. This approach links the ideas of a progression pathway, such as the UKPSF, with that of representation of reflective practice in a way that engages and enhances scholarship. It expands the concept of reflective practice in a professional context to go beyond the individual or introspective, the retrospective, the model-bound, and simple reporting of events, by incorporating elements of professional narrative. The personal is the starting point, which then, through the process of drawing on professional narrative approaches, takes the experience and the learning gained from it, and analyses and evaluates it to produce a written reflection. A professional narrative that presents a synthesis of its impact on the speech and language therapist's practice and describes how each practitioner has engaged with, and realised in their work, key dimensions of professional practice. Within occupational therapy, Bannigan and Moores' (2009) model links reflective practice and evidence-based practice with professional thinking. It highlights the importance of articulating and sharing knowledge, and focuses on the significant advantages of discourse on learning:

> Sharing ideas with others provides an opportunity to test out new learning, whereby the ideas will be validated or challenged. Having our ideas scrutinised is important because a key criticism of reflective practice is the danger of it becoming "self-referential, inward-looking and uncritical … (Boud and Walker, 1998, p.193). Sharing with others ensures that professional thinking does not become a self-validating process. Bannigan and Moores (2009, p.347)

propose a model of professional thinking integrating reflective practice and evidence-based practice.

The model describes the potential outcomes on future practice of such a collaborative, research-minded approach to reflective practice as being either: an affirmation of practice; a stimulus for the development of new perspectives; a change in practice; or an impetus to research. Other professions such as teaching also recognise the fundamental value of what are called 'knowledge communities'. Olson and Craig (2009) describe the development of teacher knowledge and how professional identity can be nurtured and negotiated within these collaborative environments: "... individuals can tentatively articulate how they are making sense of situations, explain their own actions and examine their stories in concert with others… [and] for individuals' narrative ... to be articulated, examined and confirmed, expanded or revised in light of others' experience and others' reflections and responses to our experiences" (p.670).

Through the dual mechanisms of critical reflective practice and the getting and receiving of feedback, opportunities can be identified to extend the impact of reflective practice to collaborative learning or research opportunities, which may then lead to greater output as the impact of such collaborations move towards service level, institutional or organisational change.

Approaches to reflection can adopt a predominantly competency-based approach under which skills and development are often viewed as quantifiable and, as such, subject to continual review and measurement according to externally imposed criteria and competencies. It is argued that true reflective practice should not be confined to skill- and competency-based issues, nor to reliance on models or frameworks for reflection. Such an approach runs the risk of fostering a 'product' view of reflection rather than acknowledging the process of development of professional knowledge and identity. "It could be argued that reflective practice is not one thing, nor a particular skill, but is constituted by a range of ideas whose aim is to foster a *critical orientation* to one's own professional practice" (Lea, 1997, p.2).

Such an approach to reflective practice is best understood "as a process of meta-cognition that functions to improve the quality of thought and action and the relationship between them. When understood in this light… reflection becomes 'critical reflection'. It *generates* learning (articulating questions, confronting bias, examining causality, contrasting theory with practice, pointing to systemic issues), *deepens* learning (challenging simplistic conclusions, inviting alternative perspectives, asking "why" iteratively), and *documents* learning (producing tangible expressions of new understandings for evaluation)" (Ash and Clayton, 2009, p.27), and results in learning that is transformative.

Excerpt from student work:

> At the beginning of this process, I firmly believed that process-driven learning lacked scaffolding from which to build ideas. Everything I have presented in this assignment has been learnt during its preparation. I can therefore only conclude that there had to be scaffolding present in the way things have been taught and in my independent learning, but that it was invisible to my product-constrained eye. Through using a new approach (process-based learning), I have become aware of things that were not apparent from my old product-orientated perspective. If I could not facilitate constructive change in myself, I would never be able to facilitate it in anyone else.

The development of professional identity is a process, a journey, a never-ending dynamic experience, which is experienced differently by each speech and language therapist. We hope through writing this book to have put down some markers towards a map of how we conceptualise the profession – which may aid others in the discovery process. As in the title of a book by Horton and Freire (1990) which adapted the translated words of the poet Antonio Machado – "we make the road by walking".

Judith Butler in her blog (2009) talks about the well-seasoned speech and language pathologist as having "walked down many paths, tripped on her own feet, lost her way, read guidebooks, looked to the stars for direction, retraced her steps, and chatted with many other travellers". This we have done too and share these experiences with you. But we acknowledge as she does, that everyone walking makes their own way.

> Change will not come if we wait for some other person, or if we wait for some other time. We are the ones we've been waiting for. We are the change that we seek.
>
> (Obama, 2008)

References

Ash, S.L. & Clayton, P.H. (2009) Generating, deepening, and documenting learning: The power of critical reflection in applied learning. *Journal of Applied Learning in Higher Education*, 1, 25–48.

Bannigan, K. & Moores, A. (2009) A model of professional thinking: Integrating reflective practice and evidence based practice. *Canadian Journal of Occupational Therapy*, 76(5), 342–350.

Bondi, L., Carr, D., Clark, C. & Clegg, C. (2011) *Towards Professional Wisdom: Practical Deliberation in the People Professions*. Farnham: Ashgate Publishing.

Boud, D. & Walker, D. (1998) Promoting reflection in professional courses: the challenge of context. *Studies in Higher Education*, 23(2), 191–206.

Butler, J. (2009) butlerspeechtherapy.blogspot.com/2009/.../walking-together-and-apart

Clark, A. & Moss, P. (2001) *Listening to Young Children: The Mosaic Approach*. London: National Children's Bureau for the Joseph Rowntree Foundation.

Dall'Alba, G. (2009) Learning professional ways of being: Ambiguities of becoming. *Educational Philosophy and Theory*, 41, 34–45.

Freire, P. (2002) Challenging the 'banking' concept of education. In A. Pollard (Ed.), *Readings for Reflective Teaching*. London: Continuum.

Glaser, B.G. & Strauss, A.L. (2012) *The Discovery of Grounded Theory: Strategies for Qualitative Research*. New Jersey: Transaction Publishers.

Health and Care Professions Council Standards of Education and Training. http://www.hcpc-uk.org/assets/documents/1000295EStandardsofeducationandtraining-fromSeptember2009.pdf

Health and Care Professions Council Standards of Education and Training. http://www.hpc-uk.org/assets/documents/10000529Standards_of_Proficiency_SLTs.pdf

Hinckley, J.J. (2008) *Narrative-based Practice in Speech-Language Pathology: Stories of a Clinical Life*. Abingdon: Plural Publishing.

Horton, M. & Freire, P. (1990) *We Make the Road by Walking: Conversations on Education and Social Change* (edited by Brenda Bell, John Gaventa and John Peters). Philadelphia: Temple University Press.

Jasper, M. (2006) *Professional Development, Reflection and Decision-making*. Oxford: Blackwell Publishing.

Kirschenbaum, H. & Henderson, V. (1990) *The Carl Rogers Reader*. NY: Houghton Mifflin.

Kovarsky, D., Kimbarow,M. & Maxwell, M. (1999) The construction of incompetence during group therapy with traumatically brain injured adults. In: D. Kovarsky, J.F. Duchan and M. Maxwell (Eds), *Constructing (In)Competence: Disabling Evaluations in Clinical and Social Interaction*, pp.313–342). Mahwah, NJ: Erlbaum.

Kronenberg, F., Pollard, N. & Sakellariou, D. (2011) *Occupational Therapies Without Borders. Volume 2, Towards an Ecology of Occupation-based Practices*. Edinburgh: Churchill Livingstone/Elsevier.

Lea, J. (1997) Unpublished teaching resource. Canterbury Christ Church University.

Lingard (2008) http://www.bmj.com/content/337/bmj.39602.690162.47

McGuinness, C. (2005) Teaching thinking: Theory and practice. *British Journal of Educational Psychology, Special Monograph Series, Pedagogy - Learning for Teaching*, 3, 107–127.

Norcross, J.C. (Ed.) (2011) *Psychotherapy Relationships that Work*, 2nd ed. New York: Oxford University Press.

Obama, B. (2008) Speech on Super Tuesday February 5, 2008 http://www.nytimes.com/2008/02/05/us/politics/05text-obama.html?pagewanted=print transcript

Olson M.R. & Craig, C.J. (2009) "Small" stories and meganarratives; Accountability in balance. *Teachers College Record*, 111(2), 547–572.

UK Professional Standards Framework (UKPSF) http://www.heacademy.ac.uk/ukpsf

Rolfe, G., Jasper, M. & Freshwater, D. (2010) *Critical Reflection in Practice: Generating Knowledge for Care*, 2nd ed. Basingstoke: Palgrave Macmillan.

Royal College of Speech and Language Therapists Curriculum guidelines http://www.rcslt.org/about/work_with_universities/curriculum_guidelines

Quality Assurance Agency. http://www.qaa.ac.uk/en/Publications/Documents/Subject-benchmark-statement-Health-care-programmes---Speech-and-Language-Therapy.pdf

Simmons-Mackie, N. & Damico, J.S. (1999) Social role negotiation in aphasia therapy: Competence, incompetence, and conflict. In D. Kovarsky, J.F. Duchan and M. Maxwell (Eds) *Constructing (In)Competence: Disabling Evaluations in Clinical and Social Interaction*, pp.313–342. Mahwah, NJ: Erlbaum.

Weld, N. (2012) *A Practical Guide to Transformative Supervision for the Helping Professions: Amplifying Insight*. London: Jessica Kingsley.

Index

3Cs (connect/collaborate/construct) 71
6Cs (care/compassion/competence/communication/courage/commitment) 139–40
accountabilities 12, 20, 75–6
achievement motivator, McLelland's human motivation theory 182
action learning 102–3, 209–10
action plans 25–6, 101–2
Action Research 21, 32
active signalling 87–91
'addiction to giving' motivations 185–6
administrative/managerial aspects of supervision 69–76
affiliation motivator, McLelland's human motivation theory 182
age 149
Ainsworth, M. 82–3
'ako' concept 201
altruism 176, 181–96
   see also motivations
American Speech and Hearing Association (ASHA) 43–4, 66, 67, 138–9, 146, 151, 153
Andersen, L. 183–4
Anderson, C. 192, 193–4
Anderson, Harlene 70–1
angelic beings 133–4
anthropology 111–14
antibiotics 57–8
anxieties 21–2, 28, 33–4, 44, 52–3, 65, 73–4, 84, 93–4, 97, 122–5, 144–5, 152–3
aphasia 129–40, 187–91, 193–6
appointments, families/carers 52–3
appraisals 20, 27, 55, 152–3
Armstrong, E. 187
ASHA *see* American Speech and Hearing Association
Askeland, G.U. 101
Asperger's syndrome 114
assumptions 28–30, 33–4
attachment theory 70–1, 82–91, 100–4, 111–12
attention/behavioural difficulties 84
attunement of parents 82–91, 100–4
audits 4
augmentative communication systems 95, 97, 110
Australia 43–4, 53, 138, 177, 188–9

autism 85, 114, 188
autonomy 38, 57–8, 70–6, 88–91, 98–9, 102–3, 120–5, 132–3, 136–7, 206–10
awareness findings, gender 160–1, 168–77

Bagilhole, B. 163–4, 166
Bandura, Albert 70
Bannigan, K. 208–9
barriers, speech and language therapy 53–5, 190–1
Bash, A. 129
Beckett, C. 28
becoming, the process of becoming 38, 203, 205–6
behaviour management 122–3, 149
behaviourism 112–13
being an object/becoming a subject 111–12
beliefs 2–13, 26–30, 33–7, 53, 55–6, 76, 99–104, 137–40, 146–7, 202–10
Bell, S.M. 82–3
Bercow Report (DCSF 2008) 192
Bernstein, B. 114
best practice 7, 69–76, 147–8, 205–10
Better Communication Research Programme 53–4
biases 9–10, 26, 28, 146–7, 157–77, 209–10
The Bible 127
bilingual children/therapists 143–53
   see also diversity
biological sciences 1–2, 110–25
blogs 184–5, 210
the body, spirituality 130–40
body language 74–5, 81–104, 133–6
Bondi *et al* (2011) 4–5, 184, 186, 202–3
Bowen, C. 151–2
Bowlby's attachment theory 82–3
Boyd, S. 164
the brain 85–6, 90–1, 110–13, 129–40
brain damage 110, 114, 129–32, 133–4, 187–91, 193–6
Brante, T. 5–6
Brinkmann, S. 132
Bronfenbrenner's ecological models 30–1
Bruner, J. 112
burnout dangers 73–4, 182, 190–1
Butler, Judith 210
Byrne, N. 161–3, 182–3, 184

Caesar, L. 152
Canada 138, 188–9
Canadian Model of Occupational Performance (CAOT) 138

careers advisers, gender 159–62, 165–7
carers 34, 52–8, 70–1, 82–4, 103–4, 111–25, 135–40, 185–96
  see also families; parents
  intervention decisions 52–8
caring concepts 194–6
Carr, W. 31
case histories 112–13, 116, 136–7, 191
Cash, K. 129
challenges to received wisdom 1–13, 20, 30–5, 76, 99–104, 176–7, 202–10
change 33–40, 65–76, 90–1, 97, 101–4, 148–9, 182–4, 192–4, 206–10
Changing Care, Improving Quality (NHS 2013) 193–4
chaos illness stories 134–6
chaplains 128, 130, 139–40
charities 129–30, 132, 145–6, 187
child abuse concerns, gender 159–60, 163–4, 166, 171–7
children *see* paediatric speech and language therapists
civic duties 183–4
Clewley, K. 193
client-centred approaches 4, 8–9, 52–8, 98–9, 103–4, 119–20, 124–5, 130–1, 136–40, 192–6, 203–10
clients 4, 8–9, 43–58, 67–76, 98–9, 101–4, 119–20, 124–5, 130–1, 135–40, 185–6, 187–96, 203–10
  see also carers; families; parents
  dependent relationships 185–6, 187–96
  institutionalised client controls 187–8
  intervention decisions 43–58
  patient dignity policies 136–40
  power issues 182, 185, 187–96
  service user involvement 85–6, 189–96
  supervision models 67–76
clinical autonomy 57–8, 70–6, 206–10
Clinical Guidelines (RCSLT) 139
clinical practices
  guidelines 8, 139, 207–8
  received wisdom 1–2, 6–13, 76, 99–104, 202–10
clinical reasoning 4, 6–13, 76
'co-creation' 136, 193–4
co-design concepts 193–6
co-presence role of the therapist 132–3, 136
co-production practices 193–6
Cocks, N. 181–2
Code, C. 187
code switching between languages 144–5

cognitive development milestones 112–13
cognitive dissonance 33–5
cognitive psychology 33–5, 109–25, 131–2, 138
collaborative language-based therapy 70–1
collaborative learning 115–25, 202–3
collaborative partnerships 4, 12–13, 30, 34, 35, 39–40, 43–4, 50–8, 70–1, 75–6, 79–104, 110–25, 132–3, 153, 188, 189–96, 202–10
colonialism 187
comas 133–4
Communicating Quality 3 139
communication difficulties 83–91, 100–4, 109–25, 129–40, 188–96
communication model, inter-professional collaborative learning 116–17
Communication Trust 53–4
compassion 183–4
competence concepts 3–6, 18–20, 38–40, 65–6, 69–70, 85, 139–40, 143, 149–53, 202–10
  see also knowledge
Comprehensive Aphasia Test 131
conclusions 201–10
conjunctions 46
Connect UK 132, 187
consolidation, 'period of consolidation' 56–7
consultative (indirect) models of intervention 44–58, 100
contexts 3, 6, 12–13, 17–18, 20–3, 26–7, 30–2, 39–40, 67–76, 109–25, 202–10
  see also cultural issues; work...
  rarely explored contexts 3, 202–10
continuing professional development (CPD) 18–20, 24–5, 28, 36, 39–40, 101–2, 103–4, 121, 124–5, 147–8, 206–10
convenience sampling 168–77
Conversation Partner Scheme 132
conversational skills 47, 132
cooperation model, inter-professional collaborative learning 116
coordination model, inter-professional collaborative learning 115–16
cortisol 93
cost-benefit analyses, interventions 49, 58
countertransference 71–6
Coupe O'Kane and Goldbart (1998) 99–100
CPD *see* continuing professional development
Craig, C.J. 209
creativity 102–3, 129–40

Index

crime statistics 159–60
critical appraisal skills 3–13, 27–30, 35, 36–40, 55–8, 101–4, 153, 202–10
critical pedagogy 206–7
Cross, S. 163–4, 166
cry-response interactions 111–25
cultural awareness/competence, diversity 143, 149–53
cultural intelligence (CQ) 149–50
cultural issues 1–2, 3–6, 10, 13, 20, 30–2, 39–40, 53, 81–104, 109–26, 143–56, 190–1, 192–6
　see also contexts; diversity; socio…
　SLT/education overlaps 109–10, 114–25
　'swampy lowlands' of professional culture 6
Cultural Values Questionnaire 147
Cummins, Keena 74, 79–108
curriculum issues 1–2, 9–10, 11–12, 98–9, 114–25, 139–40, 146–7, 152–3, 201–2
Cushman, P. 164, 166

Dahlborg-Lyckhage, E. 166–7
Dall'Alba, G. 205
Damico, J.S. 190, 194–5, 204
decisions
　dosage 44–58, 87–91, 100–4, 115–17
　emotions 76
　interventions 43–58
deep learning 101, 103–4, 209–10
Delworth, U. 69–70
Demos, E.V. 96
Denmark 183–4
dependent relationships, motivations 185–6, 187–96
developmental levels, supervision 69–71, 76, 101–2
diagnosis 99–104, 119, 128–9, 143–5, 152–3
'difficult families' 55–6, 80
direct models of intervention 44–58, 100
disability activism 191–2
disability studies 191–2
discomfort/dissonance aspects, reflective practices 30, 32–5
discrimination issues, diversity 146, 165–6
diversity 11, 13, 28–30, 53, 143–56, 157–79, 203–10
　see also ethnicity; gender
　challenges 143–5, 147–8, 152–3, 176–7, 203
　concepts 143–53, 157–77, 203
　CPD 147–8

cultural awareness/competence 143, 149–53
cultural intelligence 149–50
discrimination issues 146, 165–6
knowledge 144–53
monolingual therapists 143–53
recruitment policies 146, 167–77
reflective practices 153
service provision 148–9
statistics 145–6, 148–9, 157–9
supervision 149–53
support requirements 152–3, 176–7
training 146–53, 176–7
doctors 150
Dodd, B. 147–8
dosage decisions 44–58, 87–91, 100–4, 115–17
　see also duration…; form…; frequency…; intensity…; interventions
　caps 48–9
　optimal doses 49–50, 87–91
　untested dosages 48–9
　video 87–91
duration-of-dosage intervention decisions 46–58, 87–91, 100, 115–17
Dweck, C.S. 33
Dynamic Assessment method 110
dynamic/complex disorders, interventions 52–3
dysarthria 131–2
dysfluency 114

EAL *see* English as an additional language
ecological systems 30–1, 73–4
education 8–13, 17–20, 50–8, 69–76, 79, 85, 97–9, 109–25, 143–5, 157–8, 183, 203–10
　see also learning; schools; teaching; training
　public perceptions 162–6, 168–77
　SLT overlaps 109–10, 114–25
　sociocultural perspectives 109–25
　video usage 97–9, 119
educational aspects of supervision 69–76
Edwards, J.K. 70–1
Egan, G. 185
emerging skills, video usage 81–104
emotions 21–2, 28, 33–4, 44, 52–3, 65, 72–6, 82–4, 93–4, 96–7, 112–25, 144–5, 152–3, 158–9, 173–7, 183–4
　decisions 76
　supervision 65, 72–6
empathy 7, 34, 82–4, 100–4, 120–1, 139–40,

157–9, 173–7, 183–4, 194–6, 203–4
  see also attunement...; interpersonal skills; therapeutic alliance
employability, paediatric interventions 49–50
empowerment 100, 102–3, 114, 139–40, 187–8, 190
Enderby, P. 58
English as an additional language (EAL) 114–16
environmental impacts 30–1, 85–6, 206–10
epistemology 17–18, 36, 203
  see also knowledge
Equality and Human Rights Commission 159
Eraut, M. 17–19
ethical frameworks 1–2, 4, 20, 28, 55–8, 68–9, 206–10
ethnicity 13, 143–53, 157, 187
  see also diversity
  statistics 145–6, 148–9
Everyone Counts; Planning for Patients... (NHS) 189
evidence, reflective practices 30, 39–40
evidence-based practice 3–4, 7, 8–9, 43–64, 66, 120–1, 186, 194–6, 202–10
  see also research and scholarship
  definition 45–51
exercises 34, 131–2
experience based co-design approaches 193–6
experiences 3–6, 23, 33–4, 76, 85–7, 90–1, 103–4, 124–5, 137–40, 167–77, 184–5, 193–6, 210
  see also reflective practices
expert models 52–3, 121–3, 136–7
expertise concepts 3–6, 121–3, 136–7, 188–9, 191, 193–6, 208–10
  see also knowledge...
explicit knowledge
  see also propositional...
  concepts 5–6, 87–8
  tacit knowledge 5–6, 76, 87–91
exploration and experimentation, key video focus points 93–7
expressive language difficulties 133–4
extending, sentence-structure/vocabulary development 94–7
extending language 87–91, 94–7
eye contact 84, 87, 92–7, 101–4
Eyler *et al* (1996) 24
face watching 92–9, 101–4

facilitated communication 187–8
families
  see also carers; parents
  appointments 52–3
  'difficult families' 55–6, 80
  intervention decisions 43–58
  'poor/non-attenders' 55–6
  video uses 79–104
feedback 21, 35, 69–70, 82, 86–92, 95–7, 118–19, 163, 208–10
  see also video
femininity concepts 158–61, 166–7, 170–1, 173–7
  see also gender
Ferguson, A. 186, 187, 188–9
Festinger, L. 33
Finlay, L. 34–5
fixing processes 195–6
focused individualised video interaction therapy 83–104
Foley, G. 73–4
Fook, J. 20, 23, 31, 101
form-of-dosage intervention decisions 46–58, 100, 115–17
formative aspects of supervision 68–9
Fourie, R. 71–3, 182, 185–7, 190, 194, 196
frames of reference 33–4
'Framework' approach of Richie and Lewis 168
Francis Report (2013) 136, 139–40, 192–3
Frank, A. 134–6, 186
Frankl, V. 131
Freire, P. 201, 206, 210
frequency-of-dosage intervention decisions 44–58, 87–91, 100, 115–17
Fudge, Wolfe and McKevitt (2008) 189–90
future orientations, reflective practices 37–40

Gallagher, Aoife 43–64
Galliers *et al* (2012) 190–1
gay men 159, 163
GCSE choices, gender 159
Geller, E. 73–4, 182
gender 13, 28, 143–53, 157–79
  see also diversity
  awareness findings 160–1, 168–77
  careers advisers 159–62, 165–7
  child abuse concerns 159–60, 163–4, 166, 171–7
  concepts 157–77
  conclusions 176–7

definition 158–9
GCSE choices 159
homosexual men 159, 163
isolation concerns 164–5, 171–7
males a criminals 159–60, 172
masculinity/femininity concepts 158–9, 166–7, 170–1, 173–7
nursery staff 159
peer support 176–7
personal interest 165–7, 169–77
professional/personal interactions with SLT 161
public perceptions of SLT 162–6, 168–77
recent research findings 167–77
research findings 167–77
safeguarding perceptions 163–4, 171–7
salaries 161–2, 165–7, 168–77
sexual orientation 149, 159, 163
statistics 157–62
stereotypes 157–79
support requirements 176–7
traditional occupations 158–60
'whipping boys' 164–5
Gerhardt, Sue 82–3
Gibbs' reflective tool 29
goal-setting guidelines, reflective practices 38–9
God 127–8, 133–4, 137–8
GPs 57–8
grammar 46, 95, 99–100, 114
Greenstreet, W. 132
Greenwood *et al* (2006) 160, 165–6
Griffer, M. 149–50
Grounded Theory (GT) 21–2, 207
grounding 21–2, 95–7, 207
group interactions/dialogues, cognitive dissonance 34–5
group therapies, paediatric interventions 49–58, 80
growth mind-set 33–4

Halliday's three knowledges 110–15
Hammell, K. 187
Hand, L. 187
'handing over' responsibilities 50–1
Hanen group interventions 53
haptic medium of signing 113
Hawkins, P. 67–8, 75, 185
HCPC *see* Health and Care Professions Council
head teachers 117
Health and Care Professions Council (HCPC) 18, 145–6, 157–8, 191–2, 201, 207–8
health professionals 21, 57, 66, 67–8, 71–2, 115–25, 127–8, 129–30, 139–40, 143–53, 157–77, 181–96
see also nursing; occupational...; speech and language...
hearing impairments 85
help motivations 185–96
Hewlett, N. 164
Hinchliff, S. 24
Hinckley, J.J. 203–4
Hird, K. 181–2
historical perspectives, sociocultural perspectives 111–13
holistic approaches 37, 121–2, 130–1, 137–40, 195–6
Holler, J. 95–6
Holmes, M. 158
homosexual men 159, 163
honesty and openness of professionals 54–5, 57–8
horizontal discourse 114–15
Horton, M. 201, 210
Horton, S. 189, 201
'how much therapy is enough' 58
humanistic focus of the profession 194–6
humanistic philosophy 1–2, 74–5, 194–6
humility, wisdom 13

i-Pads 91
identity 1–2, 10–13, 32, 33–4, 76, 94–104, 121–5, 132–3, 149–53, 203–10
see also professional...
Illich *et al* (1977) 187
improvisational character of clinical work 8–9, 195, 203–4
inclusion 98–9, 137–40
independence principle, video 92, 97–9, 102–3
individual activities
  focused individualised video interaction therapy 83–104
  reflective practices 23–30, 31–2, 34–5, 39, 205–10
inference training 46–7
influence through eye contact 92–3, 95–6
information 32–4, 57–8, 121
see also knowledge
initiation paths 9–10
inner conflicts about expert-led services 53–4

institutionalised client controls 187–8
intensity-of-dosage intervention decisions 46–58, 87–91, 100
Intensive Interaction model 84–5, 87–91
intentionality considerations, reflective practices 23–4, 35
inter-professional collaborative learning 115–25, 204–10
  see also multi-disciplinary interactions
internalised social language 111, 113
International Association of Logopaedics and Phoniatrics (IALP) 152–3
interpersonal skills 7, 28–30, 69–76, 97, 159, 174–7, 194–6, 203–4
  see also therapeutic alliance
interpreters 91
intersubjectivity 72–3, 83
interventions 8–10, 43–64, 79–80, 87–104, 110, 131–2, 147–53, 203–10
  see also dosage decisions
  cost-benefit analyses 49, 58
  critique 44–58, 98–104
  decisions 43–58
  direct/consultative-(indirect)/wait-and-see-(review) models 44–58, 100
  dynamic/complex disorders 52–3
  group interventions 49–58, 80
  'how much therapy is enough' 58
  initial appointments 52–5
  models 44–58, 99–104
  policies 57–8, 103–4
  recommendations 57–8
  resource constraints 48–58, 103
  responsibilities 50–1, 56–8, 104
  responsive services 52–8
  six-week packages 12
  stories 10, 47
  teaching 8–9, 48–9
  termination decisions 56–8
  video usage 87–104
introspective activities, reflective practices 26–30, 34–5, 208–10
intuition 3, 6, 76, 88–91, 202–10
isolation concerns, gender 164–5, 171–7
iterative approaches, reflective practices 206–8

job satisfaction 102–4, 181–96
Johnston, D. 137–8
joint-vocabulary principle, video 91–2
Joshi, S. 67

journeys, metaphor of journeys 1–2, 132–3, 136–40, 201, 207–10
Jungian concept of the wounded healer 186

Kagan, N. 75
Kang, C. 138, 139
Kemmis, S. 31
Keogh review (2013) 192–3
Kimble, C. 144–5
Kitchen Table Wisdom (Remen) 10
knowledge 2–13, 17–40, 50–2, 69–76, 82, 101–4, 110–15, 123–5, 144–5, 149–53, 187–96, 202–10
  see also explicit...; non-propositional...; personal...; propositional...; tacit...
  concepts 2–13, 17–20, 32–4, 50–2, 70–1, 74–6, 82, 101–4, 144–53, 194–6, 202–10
  definitions 3–6, 70–1, 74–5, 194–5
  diversity 144–53
  Halliday's three knowledges 110–15
  information 32
  nature of knowledge 3–6, 70–1, 74–5, 101–4, 202–10
Kohler, P. 152
Kovarsky, D. 194–5, 204
Kronenberg *et al* (2005) 194
Kvale, S. 132

labelling of language 87–91
ladder of participation 190
language delay 80, 110–12
language disabilities 47, 80–104, 109–25, 127–8, 129–30, 135–6, 151–3, 188
language impairment 47, 50–1, 80–104, 109–25, 129–32, 143–5, 188–9
Law *at al* (2002) 44–5
Law *et al* (2010) 193–4
Leadbeater, C. 160–3, 165–6
learning 2, 12–13, 17–20, 21–4, 56, 65–76, 80–104, 109–26, 188–9, 201–10
  see also teaching; training
  about language 110, 113–14
  'ako' concept 201
  deep learning 101, 103–4, 209–10
  difficulties 80–1, 110, 113–25, 188–9
  Halliday's three knowledges 110–15
  ownership of learning 24–6, 206–10
  processes 109–17, 124–5, 203
  sociocultural perspectives 109–25
  supervision in other professions 65–76,

104, 203–5
theory 56, 109–10, 117–18
through language 110, 114–15
transformational learning 12, 201–2, 206–10
learning language concepts 110–13
learning support assistants (LSAs) 50–1
legal frameworks 1–2, 58
Leonard, L. 166–7
Lewis, J. 168
liminal space concepts 136–7
line management supervision 65–6, 75–6
see also supervision
linguistic anthropology 111–14
lip reading 94
lisping 131
listening skills 87, 96–7, 101–4, 123–5, 193–6
literacy skills 49–50, 113, 115–25, 133
Litosseliti, L. 160–3, 165–6
Loan-Clarke *et al* (2009) 161–2
locked-in syndrome 127–8
London Deanery 150
London Special Interest Group on Bilingualism 150–1
looking away 93–4
LSAs *see* learning support assistants
Lubinski, R. 146–7

McAllister, L. 67, 160–2, 164–5
McCluskey, U. 70–1, 100–1
McCormick, Marian 1–15, 17–42, 201–12
Machado, Antonio 210
MacKenzie, Sophie 127–41
McKinsey 1
McLelland's human motivation theory 182
McLeod, S. 151–2
McNiff, J. 21–2
McSherry, W. 129
Madhani, N. 146–7, 153
Makaton Language Programme 113
males as criminals 159–60, 172
see also gender; masculinity...
management-centred user involvement 192–3
managerial accountabilities 12, 20, 31–2, 75–6
Maori concept of 'ako' 201
Markham, Chris 157–79
Martin, Deirdre 109–26
masculinity concepts 158–61, 166–7, 170–1, 173–7
see also gender
Maslow's Hierarchy of Needs 132
Matteliano, M.A. 146–7
Mattingly, C. 195
maturation 110–25
Mayers, C. 137–8
Maynard, A. 28
Meadus, R.J. 166–7
meaning 111–25, 129–40, 206–10
mediation concepts 110–25
men in the profession 157–77
see also gender
Mennen, I. 147–8
mental health services 47–50, 71–2, 98
mentors, training 176–7
meta-cognition 24–5, 101–3, 113–25, 207–10
see also reflective practices
meta-linguistic therapy 113–14
Metaphon 114
metaphor of journeys 1–2, 132–3, 136–40, 201, 207–10
Mezirow, J. 22, 23, 25, 29, 33
Michael Palin parent–interaction video model 85–6, 190
micro-scaffolding 118–19
midwifery 157
the mind 110, 130–40
miner model 132
mirroring of actions 93, 96–7, 101–4
Mitchell, David 40
models of reflection, reflective practices 35–40, 206–10
monolingual therapists 143–53
see also diversity
Moores, A. 208–9
morals 4
morphology 114
MOSAIC model 206
mothers
see also carers; parents
cry-response interactions 111–25
motivations 94–104, 149–53, 176, 181–96, 202
altruism 176, 181–96
concepts 181–96
dependent relationships 185–6, 187–96
to help 185–6
needs to be needed 185–6, 190–1
personal experiences 184–5

power issues 182, 185, 187–96
vocational aspects of the profession 185
wounded helpers 186
multi-disciplinary interactions 11–12, 17–40, 82, 100, 115–25, 139–40, 157–8, 204–10
see also inter-professional collaborative learning
spirituality 139–40, 204–5
multilingual families 113–14, 115–25, 143–53
see also diversity
Mundle, R. 135–6
Munro, E. 76
Murray-Garcia, J. 149–50

naming, sentence-structure/vocabulary development 94–7
narcissism 186
narrative intervention programmes 47
narrative reasoning approaches 10–11, 23, 39–40, 114, 132, 134–6, 140, 186, 204–5, 206–10
see also stories
National Curriculum 123
National Institute for Health and Care Excellence (NICE) 48–9, 137
'navel-gazing' activities 23
Neal, Catherine 157–79
near-death experiences 134
needs to be needed, motivations 185–6, 190–1
neuroplasticity of the brain 86, 90–1, 131–2
Neve, B. 160–2, 164–5
The New Reynell Developmental Language Scales 152–3
NHS 48–9, 66–7, 136–7, 146, 157, 159, 161–2, 168–77, 181–96
non-managerial supervision 65–76
see also supervision
non-propositional knowledge 3–13, 74–5, 203, 208
see also knowledge; personal...; professional craft...; tacit...
definition 3, 4–5
non-verbal behaviours 83–4, 87–92, 100–4, 133–6, 143–5
normative aspects of supervision 68–9
'not-knowing' concepts 71
Nuffield Centre Dyspraxia Programme 114
nursery staff 50–1, 97–9, 159
gender issues 159

intervention decisions 50–1
video usage 97–9
nursing 21, 57, 66, 67–8, 71–2, 129–30, 139–40, 157–8, 160, 165–7, 172–3
historical background 129–30
spirituality 129–30, 139–40

Oakley, A. 158
Obama, B. 210
occupational therapy 10–11, 21, 67–8, 137–40, 185, 187, 194–5, 204–5, 208–9
Ochs, E. 112, 113
Office of the First Minister and Deputy First Minister in Northern Ireland (OFMDFM) 159
Office of National Statistics (ONS) 159
OFSTED 123
O'Hagan, K. 150, 153
Oliver, M. 187
Olson, M.R. 209
oral comprehension 46–7
oral language techniques 46–7
overstimulation effects 93
overview of the book 1–2, 11–13, 202–3
ownership of learning 24–6, 206–10

paediatric speech and language therapists 43–58, 74–6, 79–104, 109–25, 128–9
see also interventions; speech and language...
intervention decisions 43–58
paedophilia concerns 166
Palin Parent Rating Scale 85–6, 190–1
Papadopoulos, I. 148, 150–1
paralysis 127–8
parent workshops 80
parent–child interaction therapy 80–1, 83–4, 85–104
parents 43–58, 74–6, 79–104, 111–25, 183–4, 189–96
see also carers; families
altruism 183–4
attachment theory 70–1, 82–91, 100–4, 111–12
common misperceptions 86
as fulcrums 85–6, 100–4
initial appointments 52–5
intervention decisions 43–58
service user involvement 85–6, 189–96
video uses 79–104
Parity 145–6
passives 46, 52

patient dignity policies 136–40
patterning/re-patterning issues 87, 89–94, 100
Payne, M. 186
PECS *see* Picture Exchange Communication System
peer support, gender 176–7
Pellegrino (2012) 127
performance management activities 20
'period of consolidation' 56–7
Perlis, S. 149–50
Perry, J. 183
persistence, key video focus points 95–7
person-centred care 130–1, 136–40, 192–6, 203–10
personal experiences, motivations 184–5
personal interest, gender 165–7, 169–77
personal non-propositional knowledge 3, 6–7, 9–13, 203, 208–9
  see also knowledge
  definition 3
personalisation principle, video 91–2
PGDip SLT 20–3
phonological awareness 114, 115–25
phonological recasting 96
phonology 96, 114, 115–25
Piaget, J. 112–13
Picture Exchange Communication System (PECS) 112–13
Pilhammar-Anderson, E. 166–7
Pillay, M. 187
placement learning 2, 201–2
play patterns 87
policies
  see also client-centred approaches
  diversity 146–53
  motivations 183–4
  paediatric interventions 57–8, 103–4
  patient dignity policies 136–40
  postmodern era 136–40
  supervision 69–76
political issues 30, 103, 120–1, 150–3, 191–2
'poor/non-attenders' 55–6
positive psychology 11, 26, 70–1, 96–9, 137, 196
positive reinforcement 96–9
positivist paradigm 3–4
postmodern era 136–40
power
  aspects of supervision 71–2
  differentials 150, 188–96
  imbalances 182, 185, 187–96

McLelland's human motivation theory 182
  relationships 182, 185, 187–96, 203–4
PowerPoint presentations 21
practice, received wisdom 1–2, 6–13, 32, 99–104
practitioner-led research 22
pragmatics 27–8, 47–8, 114
  therapy 47–8
  of values 27–8
pre-registration programmes 20, 71, 72–3, 138–9, 146–53, 191, 201, 205–6
prejudices 9–10, 26, 28, 146–7, 157–77, 209–10
presentations 101–2
priorities 191–6, 206–10
private sector, motivations 183–4
Prizant, B. 95
problematic aspects of reflection 17–20, 21–3, 35, 38–40, 208–9
procedures
  see also regulations
  critique 101–4
process of becoming 38, 203, 205–6
process/product contrasts, reflective practices 24–6, 27–30, 38–40, 203, 206, 209–10
Procter, B. 68–9
product/process contrasts, reflective practices 24–6, 27–30, 38–40, 203, 206, 209–10
professional artistry 4, 6
professional conflicts, paediatric interventions 53–4, 55–8
professional craft non-propositional knowledge 3–13, 203, 208
  see also knowledge; tacit...
  concepts 3–8
  definition 3, 4–5
professional frameworks 1–2, 32, 183–96, 202–10
professional identity 1–2, 10–13, 32, 33–4, 76, 99–104, 121–5, 182–96, 202–10
  definition 10–11, 205
  received wisdom 1–2, 10–13, 76, 99–104, 202–10
propositional knowledge 3–13, 74
  see also knowledge
  concepts 3–9
  definition 3–4, 6
protectionism 11
protoconversation, non-verbal behaviours

83–4
provocative ideas 2–3
Psycholinguistic Assessment of Language Processing in Aphasia 131
psychology 1–2, 7, 17–18, 33–5, 50–1, 55–6, 69–76, 82, 85–6, 109–25, 131–2, 138–40, 185–6
psychoneurobiological processes, video 85–6, 90–1
psychotherapy 73–4, 82, 185–6, 203
public perceptions, SLT 162–6, 168–77
public service motivation (PSM), definition 183–4
purpose in life 129–40

QAA *see* Quality Assurance Agency
qualitative research 21–2, 167–77
Quality Assurance Agency (QAA) 19, 201
quality-of-life 129, 132–3
quantitative research 21–2
quest illness stories 134–6, 140
questioning beliefs/values 2–13, 27, 34–7, 55–6, 76, 99–104, 202–10

Raddon, A. 36
randomised controlled trials (RCTs) 47–58
rarely explored contexts 3, 202–10
RCSLT *see* Royal College of Speech and Language Therapists
RCTs *see* randomised controlled trials
'readiness for therapy' 54–5
reading comprehension and inferencing skills 46–7, 85–6, 115–16
reasoning 4, 6–13, 23, 39–40, 76
recasting, sentence-structure/vocabulary development 87–91, 94–7
received wisdom
  challenges 1–13, 20, 30–5, 76, 99–104, 176–7, 202–10
  reflective practices 18–20, 21–40, 76
  speech and language therapy and professional identity 1–13, 76, 99–104, 202–10
reciprocal learning 201–2, 205–10
recommendations, paediatric interventions 57–8
recruitment policies, diversity 146, 167–77
reflective practices 2, 9–13, 17–42, 43–4, 71–6, 79–80, 81–104, 118, 120–3, 153, 186, 192–3, 196, 201–10
  see also self...
  collaborative partnerships 30, 34, 35, 39–40, 79–80, 101–4, 192–3, 205–10
  conclusions 38–40, 201–10
  contexts 17–18, 20–3, 26–7, 30–2, 39–40, 101–4, 206–10
  definitions 17–23, 27–8, 30–2, 38–40, 206–10
  discomfort/dissonance aspects 30, 32–5
  diversity 153
  evidence 30, 39–40
  forms 18, 27–8, 35–40, 206–10
  future orientations 37–40
  individual activities 23–30, 31–2, 34–5, 39, 205–10
  intentionality considerations 23–4, 35
  introspective activities 26–30, 34–5, 208–10
  iterative approaches 206–8
  models of reflection 35–40, 206–10
  problematic aspects 17–20, 21–3, 35, 38–40, 208–9
  product/process contrasts 24–6, 27–30, 38–40, 203, 206, 209–10
  received wisdom 18–20, 21–40, 76
  retrospective stances 23, 37–40, 208–10
  student work excerpts 25–6, 28–30, 33–4, 36–8, 206–7, 210
  supervision 71–2, 74–6, 101–2, 186, 196, 204–5
  transactional face 27–30
  transformative face 27–30, 33–4, 72, 111–12
  video 101–4
regulations 1–2, 20, 82–5, 101–4, 157, 191–2, 201–2, 207–8
  see also procedures; self...
  critique 101–2
rehabilitation 13, 187–96
reinforcement circles 96–9
Relationship Development Intervention interactionalist model 84–5
religion 127–41, 149, 182, 183–4, 185
  see also spirituality
Remen, Rachel Naomi 10, 195–6
repair
  see also resilience
  key video focus points 95–7
repeating, sentence-structure/vocabulary development 94–7, 101–4, 112–13
reports 99, 136, 139–40, 192–3
research partners, catching/developing/propagating emerging skills using video 81–104

research and scholarship 3–6, 8–9, 20, 32, 44–5, 57–8, 81–104, 167–77, 190–1, 206–10
  see also evidence-based practice
  propositional knowledge 3–6, 8–9
resilience 12, 65–6, 70–6, 83–4, 96–9, 103–4
  definition 96
resistance
  to being given help 186
  to change 38, 192–3
resource constraints, paediatric interventions 48–58, 103
respect 57, 71, 80–1, 93, 103–4, 151–3, 182–3
responsibilities 50–1, 56–8, 104, 136–40, 169–77, 194–6
responsive services, paediatric interventions 52–8
restitution illness stories 134–6
restorative aspects of supervision 68–9
retrospective stances, reflective practices 23, 37–40, 208–10
reviews
  paediatric interventions 51–2, 54–8
  supervision videos 75
reward systems 112–13
rhetoric aspects, service user involvement 192–3
Riddell, S. 157
risk management 12, 75–6
Ritchie, J. 168
Roberts, J. 193
Robson, Begum and Locke (2003) 192–3
Rogers' influences 204
roles of speech and language therapists 2–3, 12–13, 43–8, 55–8, 74–5, 79–80, 97–104, 113, 114–17, 118–25, 128–31, 132–40, 143–5, 157–8, 173–7, 181–96, 201–10
Rolfe *et al* (2010) 32, 33, 208
Ross, L. 129–30
routines, teachers 122–3
Royal College of Speech and Language Therapists (RCSLT) 18–19, 35, 43, 65, 145–7, 152–3, 191–2, 201–2
Ryan, S. 76
Ryde, M. 150

safeguarding perceptions, gender 163–4, 171–7
salaries 161–2, 165–7, 168–77, 183–4
Saxton (2005) 94–5
scaffolding theory 87–104, 113–14, 118, 210

SCERTS interactionalist model 84–5
Schieffelin, B. 112, 113
Schön, D. 6, 101
schools 44–5, 50–8, 85, 97–9, 114–25, 159–77, 209–10
  see also teaching
  critique 98–9
  GCSE choices and gender 159
  gender issues 159–77
  public perceptions 162–4, 168–77
  roles of teachers 118–19
  SLT/education overlaps 109–10, 114–25
  video usage 97–9, 119
Schore, A. 85–6, 93
SCIP *see* Social Communication Intervention Project
segregation 98–100
the self 12, 21–2, 24–32, 35, 70–2, 82–4, 93–4, 97–9, 101–4, 130–40, 149–53, 182–4, 185–6
  see also professional identity; reflective practices
self-acceptance 132–3
self-actualisation needs 132, 134–6
  see also spirituality
self-assessments 24–30, 101–2, 149–53, 206–10
self-awareness 12, 21–2, 24–6, 27–30, 70–2, 73–4, 101–4, 114, 132–3, 149–53, 182–4, 186, 203–10
self-calm 93
self-confidence 82–5, 88–91, 93–4, 96–9, 100, 122, 143–53, 193–6, 203, 205–10
self-efficacy 70–1, 203
self-esteem 49–50, 97–9, 103–4, 185–6, 193–6
self-identity 94–104, 149–53, 191–2
self-image 12, 32, 98–9
self-management 27–30, 203–10
self-regulation 85–7, 91, 93–9
self-sacrifice 183–4
self-worth 185–6, 193–6, 203–10
SEN *see* special educational needs
sentence structure development 94–7
sentence-combining intervention approaches 46
sentence-construction intervention approaches 46
'service' concepts 181–200, 204–10
  see also motivations; speech and language therapists
service delivery 12–13, 20, 45–58, 81–104,

148–9, 181–200, 203–10
  concepts 52–8, 98–104, 203–4
  critique 52–8, 98–104, 203–4
  ideal models 102–3
  initial appointments 52–5
  inner conflicts about expert-led services 53–4
'service provider' 194–6
service user involvement
  definitions 191–2
  power relations 85–6, 189–96
serving processes 195–6
SETs *see* Standards of Education and Training
seven-eyed supervision model 67–76
Sex Discrimination Act 1975 157
sexual orientation 149, 159, 163
shape-coding techniques 46
shared ideas 208–10
'shared vocabulary' 90–1
Shohet, R. 67–8, 75, 185
sign language 110
signs 110, 113
silence, key video focus points 92–7, 101, 102–3
Simmons-Mackie, N. 190, 194–5, 204
Simpson, S. 65–6
six-week packages, interventions 12
The Skilled Helper (Egan) 185
skills 3–13, 27, 31–2, 35, 36–40, 69–76, 79–104, 121–5, 153, 159, 174–7, 182–96, 206–10
  see also interpersonal...; listening...
  video usage 79–104
Skovholt, T. 1
Skype 102
SLI *see* specific language impairment
SLTAs *see* speech and language therapy assistants
smartphones 91
Social Care Institute for Excellence (SCIE) 191–2
social class 28
Social Communication Intervention Project (SCIP) 47
social isolation, paediatric interventions 49–50
social media 102–3, 160–1
social model 4–6
social workers 76, 184, 194–5
socio-economic groups 81–2
sociocultural perspectives 12–13, 17–18, 30–2, 91–2, 101–4, 109–26, 143–53
  see also cultural...
  concepts 109–25, 143–53
  definition 110–13
  inter-professional collaborative learning 115–25
  learning 109–25
  SLT/education overlaps 109–10, 114–25
socioeconomic class 149–50
sociology 17–18, 110–12
solution-focused therapy 70–1
Sonia/Ron story, video uses 80–1
SOPs *see* Standards of Proficiency
the soul 127–41
SPA *see* Speech Pathology Australia
Sparks, C. 65–6
special educational needs (SEN) 51, 114–15, 117–18
specific 'diagnosis' 99–104
specific language impairment (SLI) 50–1, 143–5
speech language and communication needs (SLCN) 109–25
speech and language therapists 2–3, 12–13, 43–58, 65–104, 113, 114–17, 118–25, 128–40, 143–53, 157–77, 181–96, 201–12
  see also motivations
  altruism 176, 181–96
  co-presence role of the therapist 132–3, 136–40
  honesty and openness of professionals 54–5, 57–8
  intervention decisions 43–58
  monolingual therapists 143–53
  NHS 48–9, 66–7, 136–7, 146, 157, 159, 161–2, 168–77, 181–96
  power issues 71–2, 182, 185, 187–96, 203–4
  professional conflicts 53–4, 55–8
  roles 2–3, 12–13, 43–8, 55–8, 69–80, 97–104, 113, 114–17, 118–25, 128–31, 132–40, 143–5, 157–8, 173–7, 181–96, 201–10
  salaries 161–2, 165–7, 168–77, 183–4
  teachers 114–25
speech and language therapy assistants (SLTAs) 50–1
speech and language therapy (SLT) 1–15, 18–40, 43–58, 65–78, 99–104, 118–25, 127–41, 157–79, 181–96, 201–12
  see also diversity; gender; interventions; spirituality; supervision; video

barriers 53–5, 190–1
common misperceptions 86
conclusions 201–10
definition 13, 43–5, 100–1, 103, 118–19, 129–30, 157–8, 185, 194–5
education overlaps 109–10, 114–25
historical background 44–5, 50–1, 129–30, 131–2
'how much therapy is enough' 58
parents as fulcrums 85–6, 100–4
public perceptions 162–6, 168–77
received wisdom 1–13, 76, 99–104, 202–10
sociocultural perspectives 109–25
Speech Pathology Australia (SPA) 43–4, 139
spelling 116–25
Spillers *et al* 2009 138
the spirit 127–41
spirituality 12, 127–41, 204–5
definitions 127–9, 137–8
facets 137
multi-disciplinary interactions 139–40, 204–5
nursing 129–30
occupational health 137–9
in other healthcare professions 137–40
WHOQOL-SRPB Group 137
spontaneous recovery 131–2
standardised tests for English-speaking children 144–5, 152–3
Standards of Education and Training (SETs) 207
Standards of Proficiency (SOPs) 207
Stansfield, J. 147–8
Stengelhofen, J. 101
stereotypes, gender 157–79
Stern, D. 82–3, 93
Stevens *et al* (2012) 184
Stokes, Jane 1–15, 65–78, 109–26, 143–56, 181–200, 201–12
Stoller, Robert 158
Stoltenberg, C. 69–70
stories 10, 23, 47, 75–6, 132–3, 134–40, 186, 201–2, 206–10
  see also narrative...
  interventions 10, 47
Stow, C. 147–8
strengths-based approach to supervision 70–1
Stroke Association 135
strokes 12, 127–8, 133–4, 135, 139–40
student work excerpts, reflective practices 25–6, 28–30, 33–4, 36–8, 206–7, 210
stuttering 129, 131, 190
supervisees, relationship complexities 67–76
supervision 12, 20, 31–2, 65–78, 90–1, 101–4, 149–53, 185–6, 196, 201–10
  3Cs (connect/collaborate/construct) 71
  concepts 65–76, 90–1, 101–4, 149–50, 185–6, 196, 201–5
  countertransference/transference issues 71–6
  developmental levels 69–71, 76, 101–2
  diversity 149–53
  elements 67–9
  emotions 65, 72–6
  functions 68–71, 74–6, 101–2, 186
  ineffective patterns 67–8, 75, 104
  models 67–76, 101–2
  in other professions 65–76, 104, 203–5
  power aspects 71–2
  reflective practices 71–2, 74–6, 101–2, 186, 196, 204
  relationship complexities 67–76
  reviews 75–6
  seven-eyed supervision model 67–76
  strengths-based approach 70–1
  support requirements 68–76, 101–2, 103–4, 185–6
  training 65–76
  types 65–6, 68–76, 201–2
  video 74–5, 90–1, 101–4
  wounded helpers 186
support requirements
  diversity 152–3, 176–7
  gender 176–7
  service user involvement 191–6
  supervision 68–76, 101–2, 103–4, 185–6
  video 88–92, 101–4
swallowing difficulties 157, 188–9
'swampy lowlands' of professional culture 6
synchrony of attunement and attachment, video 82–91, 100–4
syntax 95–7
systems thinking 30–1

tacit knowledge 2–3, 5–6, 20, 31–2, 76, 87–91
  see also professional craft non-propositional...
  definition 6
  explicit knowledge 5–6, 76, 87–91
Taylor, B.J. 35
teacher–pupil relationships 118–19

teaching 8–13, 20–3, 36–7, 48–9, 97–9, 101–4, 109–25, 143–5, 146–53, 157–8, 159–77, 201–10
  see also education; learning; training
  'ako' concept 201
  cultural issues 119–21, 143–5, 146–53
  diversity 146–53
  gender issues 159–77
  interventions 8–9, 48–9
  pressures 122–5
  public perceptions 162–4
  reflective practices 20–3, 36–7, 101–4, 120–1
  roles 118–20, 121–5
  routines 122–3
  SLT overlaps 109–10, 114–25
  speech and language therapists 114–25
  video uses 119
teams
  diversity 152–3
  video usage 101–4
technical rational approach 4
technological platforms, video 91
termination decisions, interventions 56–8
terminology, power relationships 188–9
Tervalon, M. 149–50
Tett, L. 157
therapeutic alliance 6–13, 74–6, 100–1, 194–6, 203–10
  see also empathy; interpersonal skills
  clinical reasoning 6–7
therapist-centred models of service delivery 52–3
therapy
  see also speech and language...
  definition 4
'therapy later' groups 54–5
'therapy now' groups 54–5
Thorne, S. 111–13
time management skills 55–6
Togher, L. 187
top-down intervention strategies 53–4
traditional occupations, gender 158–60
training 7, 50–2, 65–76, 99–104, 139–40, 144–5, 176–7, 183–4, 201–10
  see also learning; teaching
  diversity 146–53, 176–7
  empathy 7
  mentors 176–7
  supervision 65–76
transactional face, reflective practices 27–30

transference 71–6
transformational learning 12, 201–2, 206–10
transformative face, reflective practices 27–30, 33–4, 72, 111–12
traveller analogy, co-presence role of the therapist 132–3, 136–40
treatment effects 47–58, 102–4, 189, 204
  see also interventions
Trevarthen, C. 112
trial and error 24–5, 97
'tripartite' composition of therapy clients 131–3
  see also body; mind; spirit...
Trotter-Mathison, M. 1
trust 25–6, 53–4, 101–4, 122, 159–60, 164, 172, 192, 195–6
truth 71
Tryssenaar, J. 185
turn-taking 83–7
Twomey, J.C. 166–7

UK 48–9, 65–7, 81–2, 115, 136–7, 139, 143–53, 157, 159, 161–2, 167–77, 181–96, 207–10
  diversity 143–53, 167–77
  NHS 48–9, 66–7, 136–7, 146, 157, 159, 161–2, 168–77, 181–96
  spirituality 139
UK Professional Standards Framework (UKPSF) 207–8
Universities at Medway 117, 183–4
'unknowability' 100
untested dosages 48–9
US 138, 144–6, 147–8, 151, 153, 188–9
user-centred user involvement 192–6
Usher, L.E. 133–4
Usher, R. 29

values 2–13, 23–4, 25–30, 34–7, 43–58, 76, 91–2, 99–104, 190–1, 194–6, 202–10
  pragmatics of values 27–8
  questioning beliefs/values 2–13, 27, 34–7, 55–6, 76, 99–104, 202–10
values-based practices 4–6, 9–10, 23–4, 25, 43–4, 50–1, 203–10
van der Gaag, A. 192, 193–4
verbalising approaches 46–7, 96–7
Verdon, S. 151–2
vertical discourse 114–15
video 6, 12, 74–5, 79–108
  catching/developing/propagating

emerging skills 79–104
common misperceptions 86
dosage decisions 87–91
education context 97–9
focused individualised video interaction therapy 83–104
independence principle 92, 97–9, 102–3
joint-vocabulary principle 91–2
key focus points 92–7
key support elements 88–92, 101–4
parents as fulcrums 85–6, 100–4
personalisation principle 91–2
questioning received wisdom 99–104
reflective practices 101–4
silence 92–7, 101, 102–3
supervision 74–5, 90–1, 101–4
synchrony of attunement and attachment 82–91, 100–4
tacit knowledge 6
teachers 119
teams 101–4
technological platforms 91
usage benefits 74–5, 79–82, 86–91, 97–104, 119
Video Interaction Guidance video model (VIG) 85–6
visions, spirituality 133–4
visualising approaches 46–7
vitality 83, 99, 102
vocabulary development 47, 94–7, 112–13, 114, 116–25, 135, 144–5
vocational aspects of the profession 185
Vygotsky, L.S. 111–12, 114–15

wait-and-see (review) model of intervention 45, 51–8
waiting lists 54–5, 100
Wakefield, J.C. 184
'walking' the road 201, 210
Watts Pappas *et al* (2008) 53
Weld, N. 73, 76, 201
welfare services 192
wellbeing 74, 129–30, 184
Wetherby, A. 95
Wh-questions 46, 76, 209–10
WhatWorks database 8
'whipping boys', gender 164–5
Whitehouse, A. 181–2
whiteness in the helping professions 150
Whittock, M. 166–7
WHOQOL-SRPB Group *see* World Health Organisation Quality of Life - Spirituality Religion and Personal Beliefs Group
Wilkin, K. 95–6
Williams, R. 151–2
Willis, P. 39–40
Wilson, E.M. 157
Winter, K. 147, 148
wisdom, humility 13
Wise, L. 183
women in the profession 157–77
  see also gender
words 113, 133–4
work context 67–76, 101, 181–96
  reflective practice 101
  supervision models 67–76
World Health Organisation Quality of Life - Spirituality Religion and Personal Beliefs Group (WHOQOL-SRPB Group) 137
wounded helpers 134–5, 186
The Wounded Storyteller (Frank) 134–5
writing 116–25, 133

Xu, Y. 165

Zen sayings 11
'zone of proximal development' (zpd) 90–1, 110

Index compiled by Terry Halliday (HallidayTerence@aol.com)